The Lewy Body Dementia Manual for Staff

Helen Buell Whitworth, BSN, MS

James A. Whitworth, LBDA cofounder

1st Edition, 2019

The Whitworths of Arizona, Mesa Arizona

LBDtools.com

***

***

The information and opinions herein should be considered an educational service only, designed to provide helpful information. It is not intended to replace a physician's judgment about a diagnosis, treatment, or therapy. Readers who fail to consult appropriate health authorities must assume the risk of any injuries. The authors and publisher disclaim any responsibility and liability of any kind in connection with the reader's use of the information contained herein. References are provided for informational purposes only and do not constitute endorsement of any website or other source. Readers should be aware that the websites listed in this book may change.

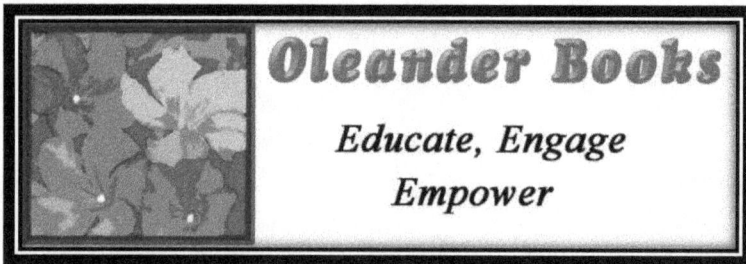

Oleander Books

Educate, Engage
Empower

Other books by the Whitworths

A Caregiver's Guide to Lewy Body Dementia (2010). An award-winning overview of Lewy body dementia and how to deal with it...."*most helpful...field guide for caring for someone with Lewy Body!*" One of over 130 five-star Amazon.com reviews.

Managing Cognitive Issues in Parkinson's and Lewy Body Dementia (2015). ..."first book I read when we began to suspect more than PD. ...calming for a new caregiver." Amazon.com review.

Responsive Dementia Care (2018). "...my favorite of the Whitworth books." "...so helpful in our daily lives." "...huge help in explaining what is going on..." Amazon.com reviews

Books by Helen Buell Whitworth

On the Road with the Whitworths: A Thrifty Couple's Tribulations and Triumphs (2015). Humorous experiences while RVing in their "new" motor home. "I loved it. It was hilarious." Reader's review.

Betsy (2nd ed., 2014, 1st ed., 2006) A novel based on Helen's family history. "*I couldn't put it down.*" Reader's review.

The Northwest McCutchens: Generation One. (2017) Facts presented in novel fashion. "*I love your books.*" Family member's review.

The Northwest McCutchens: The Exodus. (2018) The continued story of James and Mary McCutchen. "I got lost in the story and forgot to proof." Proofer's review.

All books are available on Amazon.com, LBDtools.com or McCutchenNorthwest.com

Table of Contents

Introduction

With over a decade of studying and teaching about LBD and with stressed-out dementia caregivers in mind, the Whitworths strive to present a difficult subject in an easy-to-understand manner while maintaining factual accuracy. Helen's background in nursing and psychology give her the tools to write and teach about this subject. James's detail oriented dedication keeps them on track.

Although most of the Whitworth's books are for family caregivers, this one is for care staff. Staff have many similar issues in dealing with LBD as family caregivers but there are many differences too. This book touches on both.

It started for James Whitworth when his wife, Annie, was diagnosed with Alzheimer's disease in 1999. A computer engineer, he researched her symptoms online. When he found that they matched those of Lewy body disease (LBD) much better than they did Alzheimer's, he shared this with her doctors. However, they just shrugged, said things like "Never heard of it!" and continued to treat her for Alzheimer's.

Annie reacted poorly to certain medications then considered safe for Alzheimers but even then known to be problematic with LBD. She went downhill quickly and died in 2003. James believes that the use of these drugs decreased the quality of her life and shortened it.

Even then, James knew the doctors had treated Annie the best they knew how--but few medical personnel and even fewer in the general population knew anything about LBD in the early 2000's. After Annie's death, James made it his mission to increase LBD awareness. With four other caregivers, he founded the Lewy Body Dementia Association in 2003. The LBDA is now a national organization with over 100 support groups.

When James and his friends started the LBDA, they decided to use the word "dementia" because that seemed to be the right word for the disease then. However, times have changed. "Dementia" has had and still has, strong negative connotations. In addition, it describes only one aspect of a multi-system disease and as such, is not very accurate.

Therefore, many people, including the Whitworths, now prefer "disease." With that in mind, LBD is used most of the time in this book and you can chose whether the D in LBD stands for "dementia" or "disease."

By the time James had completed his six year term on the LBDA board of directors, he had met Helen. Helen's history gives her the advantage of many aspects of the caregiver spectrum. She has been a family caregiver and a professional nurse, a nursing aide and a nursing supervisor, a student and a teacher, a researcher and a writer.

After their marriage, Helen joined James in his crusade, using her skills to help him teach and write about LBD. They welcome your stories and questions. Their contact with present LBD care partners and care staff is one of the most important ways that they stay up to date with current issues

The Support Group

The care partners, their loved ones and the care staff you will meet in this book are composites gleaned from the Whitworth's own experiences and from stories told by the many LBD patients, care partners and support group members they have known, listened to and shared with over the years.

The people below are typical of members in various local and online LBD caregiver support groups throughout the nation. This particular group is sponsored by the Anytown Senior Living Center, Anytown, USA.

Names

It may be that a person's name is the last word recognized at the close of life. Care staff know that this matters but there is some confusion about what name to use. Should it be their first name, the one their spouse and friends use? As people age and lose abilities, respect becomes more important, so maybe it should be the more formal last name and title. Or perhaps, there is some other name or honorific that means a lot to them. It all varies with the person and so that is one of the questions on the admission papers.

On the other hand, this group is a friendly bunch. They have agreed that is fine for us to use their first names as we tell their stories. They also have a good idea of the best way to address their loved ones.

Marion Peterson is the daughter-in-law of Laura Peterson, a 73 year old widow with Parkinson's disease with dementia (PDD). Mrs. Peterson, as she prefers to be called, lives in the memory care wing of the Anytown Senior Care Center. Marion is her primary caregiver and visits every day. Jonathan, Marion's son, visits weekly. Mrs. Peterson had Parkinson's disease for eight years before she began to show signs of dementia. Looking back, Marion believes there were other signs if she had known what to look for.

Janice Ashton is the granddaughter of Amelia Ashton, a 68 year old widow with Alzheimer's. Mrs. Ashton lives across the hall from Mrs. Peterson. Janice lives several states away but comes to see her grandmother a couple times a year. She became friends with Marion, who invited her to visit the LBD caregiver support group.

Norma Dupree is the 55 year old second wife of Jake Dupree, a 68 year old man with Dementia with Lewy bodies (DLB). Jake, as he prefers to be called, lives at home and a health aide comes for two or three hours a day. Jake was originally diagnosed with mild Alzheimer's. Two years later, when hallucinations began, the diagnosis was changed to DLB. Jake's children live too far away to visit more than once or twice a year.

Marie Newman is the 46 year old wife of David Newman, a 53 year old man newly diagnosed with probable DLB. They live at home with their two school age children. David, as he prefers to be called recently lost his job as a very successful financial planner because he was making gross mistakes in judgment and getting into arguments with customers.

Jenny Ellis is the wife of Peter Ellis, an 82 year old man in end-stage PDD. The couple lived together in the Anytown assisted living wing until Mr. Ellis fell and broke his hip. After his surgery, Mr. Ellis, as he prefers to be called, was transferred to the memory care wing. Jenny remains in the assisted living wing but spends most of her time with her husband.

Ellen is the much younger sister of Miss Patricia Cleary, a 78 year old woman with PD. The sisters live together in a nearby gated senior community. Miss Cleary, as she prefers to be called, is under hospice care because she has terminal cancer. Ellen first attended the LBD group because her sister talked about dementia being an advanced symptom of PD and Ellen wanted to know more about it. Now she attends because she has become friends with some of the members.

Barney Darnell is the 76 year old husband of 62 year old Hilda Darnell, who has DLB. Hilda, as she prefers to be called, lives with her husband in the Anytown assisted living wing. Barney has arthritis and sometimes uses a wheelchair.

In addition to the support group members, some care staff and the authors will also add some personal stories.

Although we use these composite characters to demonstrate LBD symptoms and behaviors throughout this book, in life no two LBD patients will have the same symptoms. As a group, they have much in common, showing similar symptoms and behaviors. Individually, each person's symptoms can be very different—early or late onset, more or less severe, demonstrated differently—or not at all. An LBD patient will seldom have all the symptoms used for diagnosis. Furthermore, response to the symptoms they do have will also vary, depending on their personality and other health issues.

A majority of LBD patients are male. An even greater majority of all LBD patients' caregivers are female. Therefore, for simplicity's sake, we refer to LBD caregivers as female, unless we are discussing a specific one. This is not to discount the many male caregivers and their female loved ones.

Overview

Before we can adequately discuss the Lewy body disease and its care, you need to know what dementia is...and isn't. While there is a lot to LBD besides dementia, it is still its core symptom. It is the symptom that causes people to confuse it with Alzheimer's or other diseases with dementia symptoms. It is often the symptom that causes patients, care partners and families the most frustration.

Of course, a good understanding of Lewy body disease and how it damages the brain is important too. With this information, you can work to change your own attitude and behavior to be more effective with what can be very difficult situations.

1. What is Dementia?

ability, skill or function: The means to perform a task.

attention: The ability to focus for a period of time without being distracted

cognitive abilities: Memory, thinking, perceptual, attention and impulse control skills used for intellectual activity.

deficit: Lower than normal

executive functions: Abilities used in thinking such as reasoning, planning, decision making, sequencing, prioritizing and generalizing.

progressive decline: Ongoing, continually getting worse.

visuo-perceptive ability: Perceptual abilities such as hand-eye coordination, depth perception and other vision-related tasks.

***

The formal definition for degenerative dementia is: "The progressive decline of cognitive abilities so severe that it interferes with a person's social, occupational and daily living activities."

Notice that this definition is for degenerative dementia. Most people with dementia have the degenerative type, which includes Alzheimer's and LBD. However, there are many dementias that are not degenerative...just not very many people have them! Notice the use of the word "dementias." Dementia is a group of symptoms, not an individual disease. In fact there are over 70 different kinds of dementia, although only a few are very common. LBD is the second most common after Alzheimer's.

Before one can intelligently discuss LBD, one must first understand a little more about what the term "dementia" means. When I first met Jim, I misunderstood the term. I thought it was the same as Alzheimer's. I wasn't alone. That's a common mistake. Also, somewhere in the back of my mind was this vision of a demented, demonic or irrational being. This inaccurate but common picture makes dementia a scary and embarrassing disease that patients and families tend to hide--and to hide from.

While someone with dementia can show any or all of those scary behaviors on occasion, the basic definition of dementia is much milder---a decline of cognitive abilities.

Cognitive Abilities

Cognitive abilities, or skills, can be divided into these categories: perception, executive functions, attention, memory, impulse control and language skills.

Dementia

...Is A Syndrome.

Dementia[1] is not a specific disease but syndrome, or a collection of symptoms, with over seventy different causes. Most of us think of Alzheimer's disease when we hear "dementia" and this IS what a person with dementia will have about 60-80% of the time. Another 20% of patients will have stroke-caused vascular dementia. Lewy body dementia, in either the DLB or PDD form takes up another 20-35% of the dementia pie chart. As you can see, this adds up to well over 100%. That's because a person may have two or even three kinds of dementia at the same time.

...May Or May Not Be Degenerative.

LBD is a degenerative dementia, as is Alzheimer's. This means that cognitive functioning gradually decreases over time. So far, neither can be completely stopped. Stroke-caused vascular dementia is not truly degenerative, although with many small strokes, the process appears degenerative. The symptoms are the result of almost immediate damage. Preventing the strokes will often stop further cognitive degeneration.

...Is Usually Complex.

Most dementias are mixtures of two or more kinds of dementias, usually Alzheimer's, LBD and/or vascular. Therefore Alzheimer's researchers claim these mixed dementias as Alzheimer's; LBD

8

researchers claim them as LBD, etc. The lack of a single cause also makes diagnosis a difficult and inexact science.

Often, a dementia will be diagnosed initially as Alzheimer's--it is after all, the most prevalent. Then as the disease progresses, LBD symptoms may become more prominent and the diagnosis may change—or it may not depending on the physicians involved, their knowledge of LBD and the medications they are prescribing. At other times, when the patient already has PD, the symptoms may be seen simply as advanced PD.

...Affects Only Abstract Thinking

Thinking abilities are divided into concrete and abstract skills. Dementia affects only the abstract thinking--the more complex skills. A person living with dementia can still do concrete thinking, which is very basic, without any extenuating circumstances. With concrete thinking, what a person sees, hears or feels is all there is. Concepts and ideas are out. Everything is here and now.

...Can Be Divided Into Categories

Various areas of the brain each control certain kinds of skills. As dementia damages that area, those skills will be impaired. These can be grouped in categories, although sometimes more than one skill is involved.

- Perception
- Executive functions
- Memory
- Visio-spatial skills
- Impulse control
- Motor skills
- Autonomic functions

These are also the categories used to discuss care and treatment.

Reasons For An Early Diagnosis

Reversible Dementias

Some illnesses such as depression, drug intoxication, hypertension and thyroid dysfunction can cause memory loss and other cognitive dysfunctions. Many illnesses can cause dementia-like symptoms. With treatment, these symptoms usually decrease or disappear. The earlier the treatment, the better the success.

Some medical conditions cause a dementia that is reversible with surgery. Hydrocephalous (water on the brain) has LBD like symptoms including dementia and motor dysfunctions. With the insertion of a shunt, the pressure on the brain decreases and so does the dementia. Brain tumors can also cause dementia symptoms that disappear with the removal of the tumor. In both cases, the earlier the treatment, the more likely it is that the dementia will be totally reversed.

Some dementias can be stopped although already present symptoms may not be reversible. For example vascular dementia, caused by repeated small strokes, can be stopped if the reason for the strokes can be stopped.

Appropriate Medication And Care

While most dementia patients tend to respond well to cognition medications, those with LBD tend to respond negatively to traditional antipsychotic and anxiety medications--and some Parkinson's drugs. An early diagnosis of LBD will alert the patient's physician to avoid medication proven dangerous to those with this disease, thus increasing their chances of a better quality of life for a longer time.

Care partners and family members do better when they can identify the reasons for their loved one's dementia-related behavior. In fact, any caregiver who understands how dementia works will be able to provide better patient care, will be less frustrated and will trigger fewer behaviors in their loved one

2. Emotions

emotion: A chemical response to a change that is hard-wired and instinctive, as distinguished from reasoning or knowledge.

feelings: Mental associations and reactions to an emotion that are personal, acquired through experience.

residual feelings: Those feelings left in the emotional memory from a previous experience.

***

Emotions are so closely connected to what happens in the brain that you need to know how they function before you can understand how a damaged brain functions. All information gathered by the senses passes the emotional control center before it is processed further. Thus, when a person's complex thinking abilities are damaged, those emotions determine the final thought. We think of emotions and feelings interchangeably but actually, emotions occur first and then, within seconds, we each put our own spin on it, depending on our own experiences. That feeling is what gets passed on to the brain's cognitive areas.

To get a first-hand experience of how emotions control our thinking, think about a time when you were startled. Perhaps a clerk suddenly appeared behind you when you were browsing the clothing rack.

- The startle is your brain's initial response to the experience. The sudden, unexpected event triggered your emotional center to send you a warning: "Danger! Run!" This is as it should be. We need to be warned quickly so that if something is truly wrong, we can react appropriately.
- Then the information traveled to your brain where you evaluated the situation, found it safe and rejected the warning.
- You laughed and thanked the clerk for her help. You replaced your original burst of fear with positive feelings more appropriate for the situation.

A person living with LBD gets the normal emotional warning because the area that controls emotions is usually intact. But then, they are stuck with that. They are also still able to assign a feeling to the emotion, using their emotional memory which lasts much longer than cognitive memory does. However, with impaired thinking skills, they can't evaluate the feeling and shrug it off and so they stay scared.

I really blew it with Mr. Ellis yesterday. I didn't let him know I was in the room before I touched him. Now he won't have anything to do with me. - Anna, health aide

Since the first information Mr. Ellis received about Anna was a danger warning, he is now afraid of her. He sees her as an enemy, someone to be avoided or fought off. Emotional memory depends on the strength of the emotion attached. Since he was very frightened, he may remember this for some time.

Often, the emotion that triggers the first thought is residual, left over from another earlier experience. A person living with LBD who has had a bad experience with a health aide wearing red may be afraid of all health aides wearing red or even all people wearing red. Yes, that is generalizing, which they probably can't do cognitively but can still do emotionally.

As humans, we attach an emotion and feelings to anything we experience. With intact abstract thinking abilities, a person can make judgments as to the accuracy of these and move on from there. A person living with dementia often can't. Without the ability to think abstractly, they are stuck believing the first information they get about what their senses deliver.

This information is also probably going to be negative. That's because negative emotions are stronger, last longer and are more demanding of attention than positive emotions, which are more soothing and gentle.

Action: When a patient expresses fear of a trusted helper, make sure it is the person and not something about them (like the red shirt). Then if it is, that person should not work with that patient for several weeks. (Negative emotions do last a long time but may eventually fade.)

Positive emotions also last, although they are more gentle. They are less insistent and may need to be encouraged and nurtured by those around the person.

Action: Encourage family members to visit loved ones even after the person's memory has failed so much that they don't recognize anyone anymore. They can still remember the emotions connected to the visitor, the feelings of closeness, of loving and being loved.

Action: Use gentle touching and tone to elicit positive emotions which will help a patient to feel more comfortable with you.

3. Dementia Prevention

At present, progressively degenerative dementias like Alzheimer's and Lewy body disease are not preventable. You probably can't even slow them down very much. You can decrease symptoms and add quality to life but the damaged proteins just keep on adding up no matter what you do.

Drugs

Researchers are still working on finding a drug that will do away with the damaged proteins that cause these dementias. The first step was to identify the type of treatment that would work best and when to use it. Researchers now know that our best chance at "curing" these dementias is to attack the damaged proteins that cause the damage early.

The next step has been to find something besides symptoms to identify their presence. By the time there are symptoms, it is too late. Researchers are now using biomarkers to do this but they still have a long way to go before this becomes common. For one thing, more research needs to be done to discover who is most at risk--who needs to take these expensive biomarker tests and just when.

Of course, the tests aren't very helpful if there is no way to treat the beginning dementia. Researchers are gathering information about that too. They are now testing a vaccine designed to guide a patient's immune cells into producing protein specific antibodies. Then when a few healthy protein cells become damaged and turn into the kind that cause dementia, antibodies are on the job and able to get rid of the culprits before they do any damage.[2] Phase 2 clinical trials for Alzheimer's are in process. Recruiting for Phase 1 for LBD has just begun.

Hormone therapy: Estrogen appears to be strongly protective of a woman's brain prior to age 50.[3] In fact, one study found that each month a woman was pregnant in her lifetime reduced her risk of dementia by 5%! Hormone therapy in later life is associated with small risks of heart attack, stroke, deep vein thrombosis and breast cancer. However, if started within ten years after menopause, it may continue

15

to reduce dementia risk. Any woman considering continuing hormone therapy beyond age 60 should be advised of the risks, have clinical supervision and use the lowest effective bio-identical (vs. synthetic) dose.[4]

NSAIDs. Latest studies suggest that if started early enough, a daily regimen of ibuprofen (Advil) can prevent the onset of Alzheimer's.[5] This likely means in a person's 20s or 30s or at the latest, 40s. However, its action apparently targets the proteins involved in Alzheimer's. There is as yet, no evidence that it is equally helpful at preventing Lewy body related diseases. In addition, NSAIDs have their own side effects which can cause problems for the gastrointestinal tract.

Herbal Therapies

Vitamin D. There is a connection between low levels of Vitamin D and dementia although this may be attributed to the malnutrition that often accompanies dementia. Geriatric specialists are beginning to recommend that elderly patients take high daily doses along regular monitoring. Vitamin D is an oil-based vitamin and so the normal daily dose of 600 IU should not be increased without a doctor's advice.[6]

Omega 3 fatty acids. Foods rich in omega 3 fatty acids may lower dementia risk, but omega 3 supplements do not.[7] This is true for many nutrients that are helpful in their natural form but lose effectiveness as supplements.

Other Attempts at Prevention

Over the years, several compounds and herbal remedies have been suggested but few have proved to be effective. Ginkgo biloba, Vitamins E and C, CoQ10 and statins all failed clinical tests although there is still some hope that they might help if started well before dementia symptoms were present.[8]

Dementia Risk Factors

One way to work at preventing dementia is to avoid as many risk factors as possible. A risk factor is different than a cause. A risk factor is something that increases a person's chances of developing a disease, in this case, dementia. Some, like age, you can't change. Some, like the habits and choices that make up your lifestyle, you can. However, to be effective, you need to make the needed lifestyle changes earlier rather than later. Make them too late and you may be able to decrease the symptoms but you probably won't stop or even slow down the progress of the dementia.[9]

Drugs. Certain drugs have recently been shown to increase the risk of dementia even when given decades prior to the onset of dementia symptoms. These are anti-Parkinson's drugs such as Kemadrin (procyclidine), Vesicare (solifenacin) for bladder control and Paxil (paroxetine) for depression.[10]

Genetics. With LBD, the risk is only 10% but with other dementias, especially Alzheimer's, it can be higher. This is one we can't change.

Family history. This may be different than genetics because it included one's environment. Where you grew up may be even more important than genetics. You can't change what has already happened but knowledge and control of environmental issues, like air and water quality, can make a difference for those who follow you.

Physical inactivity. The more active you are, the lower the dementia risk. Researchers think that physical activity triggers the production of neuron-building chemicals. This is one you can change but you have to make the effort...and keep making it.

Poor heart health. The heart pumps the blood that carries oxygen to the brain. Its health strongly correlates to that of the brain. Vascular dementia is the most likely kind of dementia to accompany heart disease but others can happen too.

Untreated hearing and/or vision loss. These decrease sensory input to the brain, decrease mental challenge and increase social isolation. These can be fixed with hearing aids and glasses.

Social isolation. A major risk factor for many health issues including dementia. Humans are "herd animals" and thrive best in the company of others. This is a risk that can be lowered but not without effort and encouragement from others. Isolation tends to cause apathy, which makes the effort to connect with others seem just too difficult to do without some outside help.

Boredom. Humans need mental challenges to stay brain healthy. This is a fixable problem and one that can be fun to do. Find something you like doing and do it. Learn a new skill or game or improve your old one, read, teach, do puzzles, whatever. Just keep that brain busy!

Sleep problems. Your brain's janitorial service works during deep sleep. If you don't get enough sleep, fewer of those damaged, dementia-causing cells get swept out. Instead they build up and begin to cause damage. This is a fixable risk factor. Even sleep apnea can be treated more easily and comfortably and therefore, more successfully than it used to be.

Poor diet. This is another treatable risk factor. It is more about your general diet than about certain foods. The Mediterranean diet is well recommended, with lots of produce, fish and foods high in unsaturated fats like nuts and olive oil.

4. Lewy Body Disease

body systems: Circulatory, immune, skeletal, urinary, muscular, hormonal, digestive, nervous and respiratory.

environmental: In the air, water or food.

genetic: Inherited.

protein: The body's building block, used for the structure, function and regulation of the body's cells, tissues and organs.

misfolded protein: A protein that has been changed or damaged, so that it does something else instead of its intended task.

alpha-synuclein protein: A protein in neurons that assists the action of neurotransmitters.

Lewy bodies: Misfolded alpha-synuclein proteins that clump loosely together in neurons, expand and spread.

neurons: Nerve cells.

nerves: Neurons that make up a network of information pathways, used to pass messages between the brain and other body organs.

neurotransmitter: A body chemical in neurons that passes the messages from one neuron to another.

toxins: Substances known to be damaging to the body.

***

Lewy body disease (LBD) is the second most common type of progressive dementia, after only Alzheimer's disease, and yet it is relatively unknown, even in the medical field. Dr. James Galvin,[11] a leading expert on LBD, called it "the most common disease you've never heard of." He explains that much of the confusion is due to how it mimics the symptoms of both Alzheimer's and Parkinson's and thus is often diagnosed as one or the other. Early-appearing behavioral symptoms can also mimic psychiatric problems such as schizophrenia. A misdiagnosis can lead to treatment that triggers LBD's often severe sensitivity to certain drugs.

Even health care professionals who have heard of the disease may not know how to deal with it. Some care facilities refuse to take people diagnosed with LBD because they are "too difficult to handle." Others accept them but use behavior management drugs to deal with irrational behaviors--triggering drug sensitivity issues.

Drug sensitivity is one of LBD's many non-cognitive symptoms, with the drug involved often one used for behavior management. Some facilities have done their homework and do know how to care for these often baffling people. That homework starts with reading books like this one but that isn't enough. This book is only an introduction. Other books, such as *Responsive Dementia Care: Fewer Behaviors Fewer Drugs*,[12] focus on dealing with dementia-related behaviors using non-drug options. Some drugs may still be needed but these books offer suggestions for how non-drug options can decrease the amount required to do the same or better job.

Lewy body disease is an umbrella term for two Lewy-body related diseases, both of which involve dementia. LBD started out meaning "Lewy body dementia." Many now prefer the term "Lewy body disease" because LBD is a multi-system disease that affects far more than cognition.

LBD is a neurodegenerative disease. It causes nerves to deteriorate and fail. These nerves, made of a series of neurons, are the body's information transportation system. Compounds called neurotransmitters pass messages between the brain and other body organs along this internal highway.

What Are Lewy Bodies?

Alpha-synuclein is a neuron-based protein that facilitates the passage of these messages from neuron to neuron. By design, alpha-synuclein proteins are sticky. They need to be to do their job. When these proteins are misfolded (damaged), the proteins stop doing their intended job and start sticking to each other. These loosely compacted, sticky clumps of damaged protein are Lewy bodies, named for Dr. Lewy who discovered them in 1917 while working with Dr. Alzheimer. The Lewy bodies attach themselves to other once healthy proteins, turning them into

20

more Lewy bodies that in turn expand, break apart and spread to other areas of the brain.

What Causes Alpha-Synuclein To Misfold?

Experts believe that for alpha-synuclein to misfold, a combination of genetic and environmental triggers must be present in the body. It takes both. That is, there may be a genetic weakness but without the environmental trigger, a person will not develop a Lewy body disease. Likewise, a person exposed to an environmental trigger will not develop the disease unless they also have the genetic weakness. They may however develop something else that they do have a tendency for. We see this in areas where major toxins are known to be. People will develop a variety of illnesses, from allergies to cancer to dementia, each depending on their genetic susceptibilities.

An "environmental trigger" is something in the air we breathe, the water we drink or the food we eat. While the specific triggers for LBD are not yet known, factory smoke, herbicides, insecticides, smog, impure water and the chemicals in processed foods have all been suggested.

The Lewy Body Family

Lewy body disease (LBD) affects many body systems. Lewy bodies in one area of the brain expand and migrate to other areas. Their location in the brain determines the systems affected and the symptoms that appear. In turn, these and the order in which the symptoms occur, determine the name of the disease.

All Lewy body-related disorders occur with a higher frequency in men than they do in women. This is opposite to Alzheimer's where there is a higher frequency in women.

We now recognize five members in the Lewy body family although only two of them, DLB and PDD, include dementia and are under the LBD umbrella. The other three are "pre-dementia" diseases and are only touched on lightly here. However, they are covered extensively in *Managing Cognitive Issues in Parkinson's and Lewy Body Dementia* by Helen and James Whitworth.

Pre-Dementia Lewy Body-Related Disorders

Two of the following three members of the Lewy body family always occur prior to dementia. REM sleep behavior disorder, or Active Dreams, often does but can occur later.

REM Sleep Behavior Disorder (RBD) also called Active Dreams. This sleep disorder occurs when Lewy bodies in the area of the brain that controls dreams "short-circuit" the chemical toggle that causes a person to be so relaxed during sleep that they can't act out their dreams. Being able to physically act out one's dreams is often the first Lewy body symptom remembered. RBD has been known to show up 50 years prior to cognitive symptoms, although this time is usually closer to 5 years. People with RBD are at a 90% risk of developing another Lewy body disorder within 14 years.[13]

Mild Cognitive Impairment--non-amnestic type (naMCI). Also called MCI-LB. Cognitive impairment is a slight but noticeable decline in cognitive abilities. MCI-LB is when the decline involves thinking more than memory. About 80% of those with MCI symptoms go on to develop some kind of dementia.[14]

Parkinson's Disease (PD). When Lewy bodies gather in the midbrain and damage the neurotransmitter, dopamine, the resulting symptoms are connected to muscle function, speech and balance. Active Dreams and hallucinations are also common with PD.

Dementia-Related Lewy Body Diseases

There are two dementia-related Lewy body disorders, dementia with Lewy bodies and Parkinson's disease with dementia.

Dementia with Lewy bodies (DLB). When Lewy bodies gather first in the cerebral cortex, they attack and damage the neurotransmitter, acetylcholine. Resulting symptoms can include thinking errors and other cognitive dysfunctions and autonomic nervous system dysfunctions. Hallucinations and RBD (Active Dreams) are also common with DLB.

A person may show either cognitive symptoms (DLB) or motor problems (PD) first. The Lewy bodies may gather more in either the cerebral cortex or the midbrain. When Lewy bodies gather and expand in the midbrain, they tend to spread, or migrate, over time to the cerebral cortex.

Parkinson's disease with dementia (PDD). Around 75% of patients living with PD for more than ten years will develop dementia.[15] The motor symptoms of Parkinson's continue and the additional symptoms are similar to those with DLB. Because the cognitive symptoms are so similar, the arbitrary rule is that the Parkinson's must have been diagnosed for at least a year before the cognitive symptoms appeared for a PDD diagnosis. However, in most cases, DLB and PDD are treated the same.

The two have similar symptoms. Their main difference is that PDD starts with the motor issues of Parkinson's disease while DLB starts with the cognition issues related to dementia. Clinically, they are treated the same and so unless there is a need to identify one or the other, they will both be called LBD in this book.

Easy way to remember which acronym is which:

- LBD starts with an L for Lewy and means all Lewy body diseases.
- DLB starts with a D for dementia and stands for the disease that starts with dementia.
- PDD starts with a P for Parkinson's and stands for the disease that starts with Parkinson's.

The Diagnosis

objective test: One that is verifiable, measurable and repeatable.

subjective test: One that relies on a physician's opinion based on behavioral observations and reports supplied by the caregiver and/or patient.

biomarker tests: Objective tests of body processes in blood, other body fluids or tissues in response to a specific intervention.

***

The method of choice for the diagnosis of any disease is an objective test. However, tests done via a brain autopsy is the only test accepted as conclusive for a Lewy body disease. These tests have greatly improved LBD research and have added to our basic knowledge about the disorder but they are of no help to the live patient seeking a diagnosis.

Without an available objective test, the diagnosis of a disease must be done subjectively using symptoms reported by patients and their caregivers. A subjective diagnosis has its problems, since it depends on the reporting skills of the patient and caregiver and the doctor's expertise at interpreting them. The latest diagnostic criteria for dementia with Lewy bodies (DLB) includes objective tests called biomarkers. However, even they are not considered conclusive because the tests measure evidence showing the presence of the disease, not the disease itself.

5. Diagnosing DLB

In 2017, the DLB Consortium published an updated version of the diagnostic criteria for dementia with Lewy bodies (DLB).[16] It now includes several objective biomarker tests, most of which are radioactive tracers inserted into the body to be imaged by a variety of imaging devices: PET, SPECT, MCI, CT and Gamma.

The formal version of the DLB diagnostic criteria was written by and for scientists and dementia specialists with language that can often appear like gobbledygook to the average person. The criteria presented here is a reworded but still accurate version.

The criteria is divided into subjective Clinical Features (physical symptoms) and objective Biomarker Tests.

See the Appendix for an unabridged version of the diagnostic criteria. You can also find descriptions of the imaging devices used with biomarkers and an explanation about biomarkers themselves in the Appendix.

Essential Clinical Feature

There must be evidence of cognitive loss great enough to interfere with social, occupational or daily living functions.

- Obvious or lasting loss of memory may not appear until later in the progression of the disease.
- Cognitive skills related to attention, performing tasks and visual perceptions are likely to occur early in the progression of the disease.

Core Clinical Features

(NOTE: The first 3 typically occur early and may persist throughout the course)

- *Fluctuating cognition:* Mental function that varies in the ability to focus and be alert.
- *Recurrent and well-formed visual hallucinations*. Repeatedly seeing something unreal that looks very real to the viewer.

- *REM sleep behavior disorder (RBD).* Also called Active Dreams. The physical acting out of one's dreams.
- *Parkinsonism.* One or more of the following in the absence of antipsychotic drugs appears well after dementia symptoms are present:
  - Slowness of movement,
  - difficulty moving swiftly on command
  - tremors while at rest
  - rigidity

Supportive Clinical Features

Although these symptoms occur often with DLB (and PDD), they also occur regularly with other diseases as well. While they can support a diagnosis, they are not true defining symptoms.

- *Severe sensitivity to antipsychotic agents.* Perhaps the most important of all symptoms to be alert for!
- *Postural instability.* Unstable while standing; a Parkinsonism symptom.
- *Repeated falls.* Usually related to movement issues but can also be related to poor visual perceptions.
- *Severe autonomic dysfunction.* The autonomic nervous system controls the automatic body systems such as heart beat, blood pressure, breathing and bladder control. Includes the following symptoms and more:
  - *Syncope or other transient episodes of unresponsiveness.* A loss of consciousness, usually related to a drop in blood pressure.
  - *Constipation.* A backup of processed food in the bowel caused at least in part by an ineffectively functioning digestive system.
  - *Orthostatic hypotension.* Low blood pressure on rising.
  - *Urinary incontinence*. Poor bladder and sphincter control.
- *Hypersomnia.* Excessive daytime sleeping.
- *Hyposmia.* Loss of smell.
- *Hallucinations in other modalities.* All senses can foster hallucinations but audio ones are the next most common after visual ones.

- *Systematized delusions.* Well-structured, often lasting dramas built around a false belief.
- *Apathy.* The inability to respond emotionally. Lack of interest, enthusiasm or concern.
- *Anxiety.* Restlessness, worry, nervousness, the feeling that something terrible is going to happen.
- *Depression.* Feeling sad, hopeless, without energy.

Biomarkers

Indicative (Strong) Biomarkers

- A PET or SPECT scan shows signs of inadequate amounts of dopamine in cells that control functions related to several LBD symptoms.
- A Gamma scan of decreased tracer activity shows the heart muscle nerve damage usually connected with DLB symptoms.
- A sleep study confirms the presence of RBD (Active Dreams).

Supportive (Helpful) Biomarkers

- A CT or MRI scan that shows little shrinkage of the area of the brain involved with memory of facts and events supports a DLB diagnosis.
- Decreased activity in the occipital (vision) cortex via a SPECT or PET scan using the tracer FDG that may be accompanied by the evidence of normal activity in the cingulate cortex, which is usually affected by Alzheimer's.
- An EEG scan that shows slow cognitive activity with periods of increased levels of functioning.

Formula For Diagnosis

This section of the criteria presents a formula for figuring out if a diagnosis is probable, possible or less likely. As usual, the criteria writers are always careful to never say "always" or "never!"

Probable DLB

Probable DLB can be diagnosed by the presence of:

- At least two core symptoms with or without biomarkers, or
- One core symptom with at least one indicative biomarker.

Probable DLB <u>cannot</u> be diagnosed by:

- Just one core symptom even with supportive biomarkers, or
- Biomarkers alone

Possible DLB

Possible DLB can be diagnosed by the presence of:

- at least one core symptom, or
- at least one indicative biomarker.

Less Likely

DLB is less likely:

- In the presence of another physical illness or brain disorder with similar symptoms, although both it and DLB could be present.
- If the only core symptoms are movement issues that appear only after severe dementia is present.
- Neither supportive symptoms nor supportive biomarkers are included in these formulas. They simply add weight to a diagnosis.

6. Diagnosing PDD

Differentiating Between DLB And PDD

The statement below is included in the 2017 DLB diagnostic criteria:

DLB should be diagnosed when dementia occurs before, or concurrently with parkinsonism. The term Parkinson's disease dementia (PDD) should be used to describe dementia that occurs in the context of well-established Parkinson's disease.

The DLB criteria statement also recommends that in a doctor's office, the term that is most appropriate to the situation can be used and generic terms such as LB disease are often helpful. Research studies, where a distinction needs to be made between DLB and PDD, should use the existing one-year rule between the onset of dementia and parkinsonism to identify DLB vs. PDD.

However, PDD does have its own diagnosis, albeit, somewhat outdated.

PDD Diagnostic Criteria

The most recent diagnostic criteria for Parkinson's disease with dementia (PDD) was published in 2007 by the Movement Disorder Society.[17] It divides the defining features into four groups and then combines these groups into Probable and Possible PDD.

The groups are shown below, followed by a formula for using them to diagnose PDD.

Groups Of Defining Features

Group 1. Core Features

- A prior diagnosis of Parkinson's disease
- Dementia severe enough to impair daily activities in at least one cognitive domain.

Group 2. Associated Clinical Features

Cognitive Domains:

- Attention
- Executive function
- Visio-spatial ability
- Memory - recall of existing memories and learning
- Language - word finding, complex sentences

Behavioral Domains:

- Apathy
- Changes in personality and mood
- Hallucinations
- Delusions
- Excessive daytime sleepiness

Group 3. Uncertain Diagnosis With:

- A cognitive-impairing abnormality such as vascular without a confirmed diagnosis of related dementia
- Unknown duration of time between the onset of motor and cognitive symptoms

Group 4. Reliable Diagnosis Impossible With:

- Cognitive or behavioral symptoms that occur only with existing conditions, such as systemic diseases, drug intoxication or major depression.
- Vascular dementia, confirmed by brain imaging and neurological testing.

Formulas For Probable And Possible PDD

Probable PDD:

- *Group 1:* Both features required
- *Group 2:* At least two cognitive domains must be impaired. Behavioral features are supportive but not required.
- *Groups 3 and 4:* The presence of any of these features cause too much uncertainty for a Probable diagnosis.

Possible PDD:

- *Group 1:* Both features required.
- *Group 2:* Deficits in only one cognitive domain, with or without behavioral symptoms.
- *Group 3:* One of these features allowed.
- *Group 4:* None of these features allowed.

Differences

Differences in the PDD vs. the DLB criteria include:

- Drug sensitivity is not mentioned but can occur in PD.
- Only one mention of a biomarker (imaging to verify vascular dementia).
- Hallucinations are given less weight.
- Memory and language are given more weight.
- Autonomic symptoms are not mentioned but can also occur in PD.

The most important difference is the lack of a mention of drug sensitivities in the PDD diagnosis. We now know that as the Lewy bodies begin to affect a person's cognition, their PD drugs may also make cognition worse, somewhat like the way antipsychotics can. This needs to be something their physician is alert for and addresses early on. It often becomes a choice between better mobility and better thinking.

The bottom line remains that these two types of LBD have such similar cognitive symptoms that, as the DLB people note, it is useless to separate the two as far as cognitive treatment and care are concerned. Naturally, the person with PDD has additional physical care concerns due to the mobility issues involved but other than that, treatment is usually the same.

Cognitive Symptoms

While there is a lot to LBD besides dementia, it is the major defining feature. Therefore, it pays to know and understand how dementia affects the brain and how to deal with the symptoms that result.

Cognition is divided into two parts: concrete thinking and abstract thinking.

Concrete thinking is very basic. It results from input from the senses with little, if any, evaluation or cognitive filtering. It pertains only to what a person can see, hear or feel, is only in the here and now and can't get past first impressions.

Cognitive abilities make up our abstract thinking--or cognitive filtering. These are abilities that allow us to combine input from the senses with other available information, both physical and abstract, to develop ideas, understand symbols and concepts, make conscious decisions and think rationally.

These abilities usually overlap and a person often uses more than one at a time. We've divided them here into the following categories but they can be divided in many different ways.

- Memory
- Executive Functions
- Self-Control Skills
- Language Abilities

7. Memory

long-term memory: Where information is encoded for easier access and stored for later use.

short-term memory: Where current information is stored before being dropped or transferred to long term memory.

working memory: An area of high-speed short-term memory used to manipulate programs or data currently in use.

***

Most people connect dementia with memory loss. This is accurate more than 50% of the time because it is the prime Alzheimer's symptom. It is not accurate for LBD and this is an important difference between LBD and Alzheimer's.

Memory can be divided into several different types. The most common are short-term and long-term memory. Depending on the type of dementia a person has, impairment comes first in different ways to these two types of memory.

Working Memory

This is the part of your short term memory responsible for holding information available for immediate processing. Think of it as an open program in your computer (brain). LBD can impair a working memory, causing problems with executive functions, perceptions and language skills.

Transfer Issues

A person living with Alzheimer's has difficulty encoding new information so that it can be remembered in the future.

My grandmother likes to play the piano in the activity room. She can't learn new tunes but she can still play the ones she learned before she got Alzheimer's. - Janice Ashton

Mrs. Ashton can still remember what was already stored in her long-term memory. However, she will often repeat herself, not remembering what she said only minutes before.

Mom used to be the church pianist but she can't play very much at all. Once in a while, she can hit a few right notes but then she gets mixed up and frustrated. - Marion Peterson

Mrs. Peterson's PDD interferes more with her ability to extract old information from her long-term memory than it does with her ability to transfer new information out of her short-term memory into her long-term memory. She may not be able to remember how to play the piano anymore but she is less likely to repeat herself.

Task Memory

This involves the use of executive skills and long-term memory to know what part of a task occurs when. If a person living with Alzheimer's knew how to do something before they developed Alzheimer's, they usually can still do it. It is different for people living with LBD.

Hilda still believes she can drive but I think her driving is becoming unsafe. I wish that wasn't so because I can't drive either and this will make us more dependent on others. - Barney Darnell

Hilda's driving skills have become impaired but she can't see this because her judgment skills are also failing. This combination of adamant belief that one's skills are still present and an inability to see the safety issues involved is common with LBD, where task memories fade before general memories do. Hilda can still remember how well she drove but she can't recognize that she isn't driving like that anymore.

> *Action:* Don't argue. Instead, go along enough to move them in a safer direction. If necessary, use therapeutic fibs[a] or better yet, improv techniques[b] to keep an unsafe activity from happening. "I've lost the keys." "Someone borrowed that power saw." Use step-by-step guidance for necessary tasks such as tooth brushing or setting the table.

---

[a] **Therapeutic fib**: An untrue statement meant to help rather than harm a patient.

[b] **Improv techniques:** Entering the patient's reality and playing a part. This is explained thoroughly in the Whitworth book, *Responsive Dementia Care*.

Emotional Memory

The emotional centers of the brain work closely with the cognitive centers. However, they tend to last long after the cognitive skills have been severely impaired. Residual emotions, those initiated by a past event and stored in the emotional memory, are often the first information to get attached to a present situation.

We walked by this really friendly dog and Jake freaked out. He was sure the dog was going to bite him. I tried to tell him the dog was friendly. I even petted the dog but it didn't do any good. I should have known better. - Norma Dupree

Jake was responding to his first information about the dog, his residual fear from a previously scary experience with a dog. Since that is all his brain can process, Norma's information was rejected as false. In fact, her petting the dog was probably even more frightening.

Negative emotions last longer because they are stronger and more insistent but positive emotions can last too. That's why it is important for family members to continue to visit loved ones even after they can no longer remember them. They can still remember the emotions involved, still enjoy the feeling of loving and being loved.

8. Executive Functions

thinking: The process of developing ideas, opinions and judgments.

concrete thinking: That which focuses on facts in the here and now, physical objects and literal definitions.

abstract thinking: That which uses executive skills to evaluate, choose and understand abstract concepts.

executive skills: Abstract skills that allow a person to edit, compare, organize, develop and use concepts, express empathy and be self-aware.

***

Executive skills are complex abilities that allow a person to think abstractly and to organize and regulate their thinking and thus, their actions. The LBD patient begins losing executive abilities much sooner than the Alzheimer's patient does.

Abstract Thinking Skills

Abstract thinking skills allow a person to consider things that are removed from what one can see, hear and feel in the moment. They are what one uses to understand symbols, develop ideas and use concepts.

A person never loses all of their thinking abilities but their thinking becomes more concrete, or basic, as dementia progresses.

A person living with LBD usually begins to fall back into concrete thinking much sooner in the progress of the disease than does a person with Alzheimer's. Thus, they tend only to deal with what their senses deliver in the moment without any editing.

Editing Skills

Editing skills help a person review and evaluate incoming information and then, accept and use it or reject it.

Judgment: The process of reviewing all the available information and making a decision.

Problem solving: The process of working through the details of a problem.

Reasoning: The process of forming logical (true, accurate) decisions, judgments or inferences based on available information such as facts, theories or intuition.

Decision-making: The act of selecting a logical choice from available options.

Jake often accuses me of wanting to leave him. We've been married for 20 years and I have no plans to go anywhere but I can't seem to get that through his brain. - Marion Dupree

Jake's ability to think is compromised by DLB. He still makes decisions and judgments. However, they are often based on poor information because he can no longer use his problem solving and reasoning skills to test for accuracy.

Organizing Skills

Organizing skills are also called task-related skills because they are those used for most tasks, from simple tasks such as picking up a fork or filing alphabetically to more complicated ones such as driving or using a power saw.

Sequencing: The ability to organize items in a predetermined order such as the alphabetical divisions in an office file or the steps used for brushing teeth.

Prioritizing: An extension of the sequencing ability, prioritizing is the ability to organize items in their order of importance. A caregiver might prioritize their tasks and choose to leave the least important ones undone so that they don't become overwhelmed.

Generalizing: The ability to apply known information about one thing to another. If you know that a patient nods off after lunch, you can generalize that they are likely to nod off after any meal.

Planning: Considering the activities required to achieve a goal. When Anna, the health aide, gets her work assignment, the first thing she does is make a list of tasks for the day. She uses past experience to generalize what needs to be done for each patient and how long it will take. Then she sequences the tasks by when they need to be done and prioritizes them by their importance.

A while back, David lost his temper because the car wouldn't start. He was trying to start it without turning the key. And he was driving erratically even before he lost his job. I was getting worried but then he ran a red light and hit a parked car. The state took his license away and his doctor won't sign for him to get it back. He's furious at his doctor! - Marie Newman

David's difficulty starting the car had to do with organizing skills. He couldn't prioritize or remember which step came first--the key or the brake or the gear shift. The erratic driving that worried Marie showed that he had poor editing skills too. He wasn't making good judgments. The final accident happened when, no longer able to generalize from his store of general knowledge about safe driving, he whizzed through a red light and hit another car.

My grandmother kept getting lost. I convinced her to sell her car after a policeman found her parked by the side of the road, lost and crying. - Janice Ashton

Mrs. Ashton could probably still do the sequential tasks required to drive a car and she might even know to obey the traffic signals. But since she couldn't remember where she was going, she wasn't safe on the roads.

My wife Hilda used to be a vice president in a large advertising firm. Things that used to be easy, like filling out routine reports became so confusing that she took early retirement. That was two years ago. After she was diagnosed with DLB last year, we knew that was likely to change. I've been wheelchair bound for some time but Hilda and I have managed well. Now, with her diagnosis, we decided to move into an assisted living facility before it became a problem. - Barney Darnell

Hilda was exhibiting a loss of several forms of executive functioning, such as sequencing, planning and decision making which made her job too difficult to handle. Their concern about how long she'd be able to help Barney with his transferring was warranted. She will likely become unable to remember the steps needed to get him in and out of his wheelchair. The move was also a good step to take while Hilda was able to think clearly enough to see the issues and support the move. Otherwise, she could easily have seen the move from home in a negative manner.

Concept Development

Concepts are mental constructs, ideas about things that cannot be seen, heard or touched in the here and now. They are developed by using a variety of abstract thinking skills to combine, fine-tune and prune information from a wide variety of sources.

Time, money and distance are all concepts that we develop as we learn more about the parts of each one. As dementia progresses, a person loses the ability to use concepts.

David is beginning to have problems with time management. I've learned not to ask him to wait. He wants things done NOW! He doesn't seem to understand it when I tell him I'm busy but I can help him as soon as I'm through. He's quiet for a moment and then he asks me again. Sigh! - Marie Newman

> **Action:** To help a patient manage time, provide a task to do while they wait. Or set a timer which provides a moment-by-moment feeling.

Jake used to be so good with the money. He handled it all. Now it is all on me. He can't balance the checkbook. I had to change all the passwords on the computer too because he was buying the most absurd things. - Norma Dupree

Money and even numbers are concepts, along with frugality or saving. Without the ability to do sequences, counting and math become impossible. Without the ability to see consequences (another concept, based on past experiences) Jake couldn't see why his online computer buying was damaging to their finances.

Like concepts, empathy requires a person to think about more than just about what their senses deliver in the present time. Empathy is the awareness of others and how they would feel in a similar situation. Requiring complex thinking such as comparing and generalization, it fades as dementia progresses.

I spend a lot of time with Peter but he insists I'm not doing enough, that I leave him alone far too much. I'm not so well myself and I need to rest a lot. I tell him that and he says I'm being lazy. He used to be so concerned about me but now he just doesn't seem to care. - Jenny Ellis

Mr. Ellis is truly unable to understand his wife's difficulties. As his dementia increases, his world becomes smaller and smaller, until it is all about him and he can't see even his dear wife's pain.

Self-Awareness

Self-awareness is a conscious knowing of one's own character, feelings, motives and desires. It is what a person uses to know when to run and when they have time to walk. It is knowing how you tend to react to something, even your likes and dislikes.

Dementia limits a person's ability to do anything that takes conscious thought. For a person with only basic thinking, everything is a reaction, not a conscious, thought-out response.

When Mom gets fussy, I can usually calm her down by offering to play one of her CDs. She knows which ones she likes and she always picks out the same ones. - Marion Peterson

Due to the slow progress of her dementia, Mrs. Peterson still knows her own music preferences. Eventually, she may get to where she'll tell her daughter to choose for her. She'll still like the same music as before but she will be past making the choice to play it.

9. Self-Management Skills

attention: The ability to stay focused and to ignore distractions.

flexibility: The ability to switch from one concept to another, to review the evidence and change your mind.

impulse control: The ability to choose how to respond.

***

The ability to pay attention, be flexible and control one's impulses are all cognitive skills that help a person manage their life.

Attention

This allows a person to ignore distractions and stay focused. A person in a crowded room uses their ability to listen to one conversation and tune the others out. It also allows a person to follow through on tasks, to stay on track until a project is finished.

A person without this skill will be distracted easily and will respond to everything equally, which can be very confusing. They will need direction to complete tasks, especially those lasting over several sessions.

I was trying to tell Mr. and Mrs. Dupree about the day's activities. Mrs. Dupree was following along and asking questions but I soon realized that Jake wasn't. Then I noticed that I'd forgotten to mute the TV. Jake wasn't listening to it but he looked confused. Mrs. Dupree muted it and then he could pay attention to what I was saying. - Anna, home health aide.

Anna's ability to focus was so strong that at first she didn't even notice that the TV was on. Mrs. Dupree was able to tune out the TV enough to hear what Anna said. However, Jake, who lives with DLB, could not. His attention was spread so equally between Anna, his wife and the TV that he couldn't understand any of them.

Action: Limit stimuli, avoid media interference or multiple people and discuss only one subject at a time.

Flexibility

This is what allows a person to change their mind, to multi-task, to compromise or to empathize or see how someone else experiences something.

One of the things I always loved about Hilda was how she could look at a problem and see ways to fix it. If one thing didn't work, she'd try something new. And she'd just keep on, trying new ideas or changing old ones, until something clicked. Now she is so stuck. Once she gets something in her mind, that's the way it is. No matter what I say, I can't change it. In fact, if I try, she acts really hurt. - Barney Darnell

Barney's wife can't do the complex thinking required to make choices or to do the sort of problem-solving she used to be so good at. She isn't flexible...she is stuck with her first thought, whatever it may be. Since one's first thought is often accompanied by more urgent and demanding negative emotions, she is more likely to react negatively than she once did.

> *Action:* Do not try to change the mind of someone who has lost the ability to be flexible. It will only make them irritable. Instead, accept that this is their reality and work with that.

Impulse Control

An impulse is that first urge to act, usually in response to information coming in via the senses along with an accompanying emotion. Impulse control allows one to choose how to respond to these urges and when to ignore them. But without the ability to make a conscious choice, a person must react automatically and express the first emotion they experience, appropriate or not. Although limited impulse control also occurs with people living with Alzheimer's, it tends to show up much later.

David used to be able to keep his cool even when his customers were way out of line. But then, he started being irritable at the drop of a hat. Finally, on his last day at the office, he blew up and yelled at a customer he thought was laughing at him. I don't think they were but David was convinced. The customer complained and David's boss asked him to resign immediately. - Marie Newman

LBD had impaired David's ability to make rational judgments. Then his eroded impulse control was unable to keep him from acting out his hurt feelings with angry outbursts that drove away his confused and now distrustful customers.

It is not unusual for early behavioral symptoms like David's to be misinterpreted in the workplace as manageable inappropriate behavior. While such behavior should not be tolerated no matter what the reason, a supervisor with a better understanding of LBD would have required David to get a doctor's evaluation which could have resulted in a medical retirement, not a firing.

Mom used to be so patient but now she isn't. She wants everything done now. She blows up at the least sign of irritation. I just hate to see the change in her personality. - Norma Peterson

Like David, Mrs. Peterson is expressing her lack of impulse control. If she feels it, she expresses it and the result is that she does seem to have changed from a very patient person to an irritable, impatient person.

When Mrs. Peterson gets irritable, I just agree with her and sympathize with her feelings. Then we can usually move on. Otherwise, she gets stuck in her complaints. - Anna, health aide.

By agreeing, Anna lets Mrs. Peterson know she was heard. Sympathizing with her feelings allows her to feel understood. This will usually calm her enough so that she can communicate with, instead of at, Anna.

> *Action:* Remember that accusations and inappropriate actions are the disease talking, not the person. Align with the feelings if not the words so that you can get through to the person and redirect them.

It is important to remember that all of the differences between LBD and Alzheimer's discussed in this section become less apparent as the disease progresses. As more cognitive abilities become affected, the dementias will present with more similarity.

10. Language and Communication

attention deficit: the inability to ignore distractions and pay attention to a specific event.

word recall difficulties: Difficulty remembering a specific word--"it's on the tip of my tongue" syndrome."

word substitution: Substituting another word, often an inappropriate one, for the one a person means.

***

Communication is a give-and-take interaction requiring a combination of executive and motor skills. As you can imagine, LBD impairs both of these abilities in a variety of ways.

Language specific issues. Poor word recall, as when the word is almost but not quite there, can make talking difficult. When another word is unconsciously substituted for the intended word, this can sometimes be funny but can also be confusing.

Parkinsonism issues. Anyone with LBD, no matter what kind, is apt to experience parkinsonism features such as weakened facial and throat muscles that limit the ability to talk and show facial expressions.

Slow thinking and attention deficit. It is not unusual for a full minute to go by while a person processes a question or comment before they can come up with an answer. It can take even longer or become impossible if there is too much distraction, as when more than one person is talking at the same time.

Behavioral Communication

When other forms fail, behavior may become the communication of choice. Anger, combativeness and/or resistance can be common. It can be triggered out of frustration at not being able to be understood but it can also be a symptom that something else is wrong. A person living with LBD may hurt or feel uncomfortable and not know why. All they know is that something isn't right. Like a small child, they use the only tools they have to communicate this: attention-getting behavior such as angry striking out, yelling, blaming or crying.

Communicating Successfully

Tone and intensity both trigger a person's emotions. A loud, quickly-voiced message increases stress which encourages fear reactions and blocks a person's already limited ability to think. Conversely, a soft, gently spoken message triggers the calmer more pleasant emotions that allow a person's limited cognitive abilities to function better.

The senses remain long after verbal skills become difficult. Try communicating with a gentle touch, a soft guiding nudge. Smile, nod, use hand signals and gestures. Always be aware of your tone and keep it soft, calm and unhurried. Make sure your body language is congruent. Don't frown and nod, for example.

When communicating verbally, talk clearly, keep it simple with limited choices, give the person plenty of time to process and don't interrupt.

Patient, careful listening becomes an extremely important communication skill for care partners and staff as the person's communication abilities degenerate. Look for the non-verbal cues and use your knowledge of the person to make educated guesses.

11. Thinking Errors and Delusions

delusions: False, often paranoid, beliefs that can appear alone or accompany dreams, hallucinations or actual events.

systemized delusions: Delusions built into complicated dramas that can often last over time.

thinking error: A thought that has not been filtered by a person's complex thinking abilities and often results in a delusion.

***

When the ability to think rationally begins to fade, thinking errors and delusions start occurring. At first this is just an occasional thing. The person living with early LBD acts out of character now and then with odd, unexplainable comments or behavior. Eventually, this will be the norm. Care partners and staff must learn different skills to deal with the "off the wall" and often disruptive behavior that tends to accompany these cognitive failures.

Delusions occur when a person's complex thinking abilities are no longer functioning well enough to process, evaluate and judge the validity of incoming information.

Incoming information usually arrives at the brain's processing center complete with an accompanying emotion, often one left over from a previous experience. These residual emotions are especially likely to be negative because they are the most urgent, demanding the most attention. Without the tools to process this information, it is accepted as is, complete with its negative emotional load.

When Jake sees me talking on the phone, he is convinced that I'm talking to my boyfriend and we are planning for me to leave him. - Of course, that's not true. I'm usually talking to my daughter but I have given up trying to explain that to Jake. - Norma Dupree

Jake sees his wife talking on the phone and that triggers his residual fear that she will leave him and he will be alone and helpless. This all goes to his brain's processing center. If it was working properly, he'd recognize the fear as unreasonable because Norma has shown no signs of wanting to leave. But it isn't. And so he is stuck with the fear which has now become, in his mind, fact. "I'm afraid that Norma will leave me" becomes "Norma is leaving me."

These delusions can become very complex. Barney Darnell tells of one that lasted over several days and ended by incorporating a real event.

We live in an apartment that sits on a concrete slab. Hilda would see "workers" go down into our "basement" by way of a "door" under the sofa. In the evening, workers left the same way. Once, she offered them drinks before they went home. During our evening drive an hour later we saw a bad accident. Hilda became hysterical; she knew the accident was her fault because the driver was a worker she'd given a drink. - Barney Darnell

Hilda's delusion included hallucinations and real life events. Likewise, patients can incorporate violent scenes from TV programs into their delusions.

Wow! I learned the hard way to monitor Mom's TV. Exciting shows are likely to bring on scary hallucinations and delusions. When I can get her to watch something besides her favorite crime shows, she may still have them but they aren't so scary. - Marion Peterson

> ***Action:*** Do monitor all media and avoid anything too exciting. It all triggers those negative emotions and accompanying thinking errors.

Mom has started fighting Anna and won't let her near. They used to get along just fine but now Mom says Anna wants to hurt her. - Marion Peterson

Anna may have startled Mrs. Peterson and that left a residual fear in her mind that makes Mrs. Peterson view Anna as "dangerous." Since these emotional memories can last much longer than cognitive memories, it may be weeks before Anna will be able to take care of Mrs. Peterson safely again.

I used to travel a lot. I even wrote articles about some of my journeys. - David Newman

According to his wife, David always wanted to travel and write about his adventures but never was able to. They had planned to do so together after he retired from his job but LBD put a stop to that! David's residual emotions about how he wanted to travel and write became his reality when he was unable to distinguish them from fact.

Action: It does no good to explain, argue or defend against these thinking errors. Instead, join their reality and speak to the feelings. Then, once they are calmer, you can use distractions to move the action in a different, more comfortable direction.

Dealing with these issues is often quite difficult and distressing for care partners and staff alike. For more information and ideas about how to deal with the resulting behaviors, be sure to read our book, *Responsive Dementia Care, Fewer Behaviors Fewer Drugs.*

Cognitive Treatment

Treatment can be divided into drug and non-drug therapies. Neither can cure degenerative dementias, including LBD, nor is it likely that they can slow its progress. However, they both may be able to extend a person's time of clarity and their quality of life.

12. Dementia Drugs

acetylcholine: A neurotransmitter that facilitates cognition.

cholinesterase inhibitors (ChEIs): Drugs designed to preserve the function of acetylcholine.

Federal Drug Administration (FDA): The government branch that oversees the manufacturing and distribution of food and drugs.

glutamate: A neurotransmitter involved in processing information.

off-label: Used in a way not approved by the Federal Drug Administration.

***

These four medications do not cure dementia but they may allow a patient to stay home for up to two extra years before entering a nursing home. While few care staff will be involved in deciding what treatment an LBD patient will receive, all people involved in the care of a patient, caregivers and professionals alike, need to know the basic treatment choices and likely results.

Cholinesterase Inhibitors (ChEIs)

ChEIs, (pronounced "shies") are the drugs of choice for treating dementia in early and middle stage Alzheimer's. They can decrease dementia symptoms for a period of months or years. These drugs all need live cells to function. With the progression of the disease, ChEIs become much less effective in any dementia.

Each patient's response to these oral drugs is very individual, so the neurologist may need to try all three before deciding on the best treatment. However, only one should be used at a time because their site of action is the same. Using more than one may greatly increase the side effects without increasing effectiveness. The most common side effects include gastro-intestinal (GI) symptoms like loss of appetite, nausea, vomiting and abdominal pain. Motor dysfunctions (parkinsonism) may also occur.

As of 2019, three ChEI drugs are FDA approved to treat Alzheimer's. Of these, only Exelon is approved to treat a Lewy body disease and then, only Parkinson's with dementia (PDD). However, due to the way ChEIs function, it is possible that they could more effective with any Lewy body disease, including DLB, than with Alzheimer's. Therefore, it and the other two ChEIs are used off label regularly to treat PDD's sister disease, DLB. This is the process:

- The brain sends a message from one cell to another via a neurotransmitter, often acetylcholine. This compound can be depleted by both Alzheimer's and Lewy bodies but the latter's more specific targeting tends to cause more loss.
- Once the message is sent, an enzyme, cholinesterase, breaks the neurotransmitter down to stop it from sending the same message again.
- Cholinesterase inhibitors (ChEIs) work by interfering with the breaking down process, thus preserving the supply of acetylcholine.
- The neurotransmitter is rebuilt so that it can send another message. If abnormal depletion has occurred some of the preserved acetylcholine can be used instead.
- These steps are repeated over and over.

Exelon (rivastigmine). Marketed by Novartis, this drug is approved for PDD as well as Alzheimer's. Of the three ChEIs, Exelon has the most severe GI side effects. To combat this, Exelon also comes in a trans-dermal patch. Besides dealing with the GI problem, the patch can be easier to administer, especially to someone who resists pill taking, or finds swallowing difficult. Attached to a place on the patient's body that they can't reach, it also assures that the medication is being taken.

Aricept (donepezil). Marketed by Pfizer, this drug was approved by the FDA for Alzheimer's in 1994. The oldest of the three, Aricept is often the first drug chosen by neurologists. Clinical trials were begun in 2017 for a transdermal patch, with the hope that it will be available by 2020. Such patches are already approved for use in some foreign countries.

Razadyne (galantamine). Marketed by Janssen Pharmaceuticals, this drug is approved for Alzheimer's. Razadyne is a natural, i.e., non-manufactured, drug obtained from daffodil bulbs.

All three ChEIs are oral drugs that are also available in generic form. Depending on the drug, this can cut the cost by over half or more. Generic Aricept is the least expensive and because of this, is sometimes used even for PDD when cost is a major factor.

The support group discussed treatment at one meeting:

Barney Darnell: "The doctor started Hilda out on Exelon. Said it was the only drug approved for LBD patients. It made Hilda sick to her stomach and so he put her on Aricept. It does help. Hilda is almost normal. But I hear that Exelon patch is good so we are going to ask about it next time we see the doc."

Marie Newman: "David's neurologist put him on Aricept first. It did make a difference in his behavior but then he started having stomachaches. Now he's on the new generic Exelon patch but even that is more expensive than the generic Aricept was. It's working great though and that's what counts."

Jenny Ellis: "Peter's never had any trouble with his Aricept but I don't think it's working so well anymore. He's having more hallucinations. I just hope he doesn't get delusional again."

Although Exelon is the most irritating to the GI tract, any of the ChEIs can cause GI distress, as Aricept did with David. The patch is actually less expensive than the oral drug but Exelon and its generic are both more expensive than Aricept in its generic form. All ChEIs lose their effectiveness as dementia progresses, as they did with Mr. Ellis. It probably wouldn't do any good to try another one since his LBD is in a later stage.

Norma Dupree: "Jake's been through them all. He's on Razadyne now. I'm glad they've got a generic for it too. I'd hate to think what our drug bill would be without that. A lot of Jake's drug costs come out of our own budget. Now if they'd only have generics of all the other drugs Jake's on!"

NMDA Receptor Antagonist

Namenda (memantine). Marketed by Forest Laboratories, Namenda is approved for moderate to severe Alzheimer's. This drug's action is to preserve the amount of glutamate, a chemical that affects storing, processing and retrieving information. Namenda is seldom effective alone for LBD. However, because it works with a different chemical, Namenda can be used with a ChEI. Added to the drug cocktail when a ChEI appears to be failing, this drug often extends the length of time a ChEI is effective and in particular, improves awareness.

Namenda's mild to moderate side effects include fatigue, pain, increases in blood pressure, dizziness, headache, constipation, vomiting, back pain, confusion, drowsiness, hallucinations, coughing and difficulty breathing.

Mom just got put on Namenda, in addition to Exelon. I'm really impressed! She isn't having nearly as many hallucinations as she did have and I think her mind is much clearer. - Marion Peterson

David is on his third cognition med...and he's taking drugs for his behavior issues and his Active Dreams. And now his neurologist says she wants to try adding Namenda. What next? Sometimes, I feel like his neurologist is just throwing darts. Whatever medicine the dart hits, that's what she prescribes. - Marie Newman

Medicating for LBD is an experimental process because no two patients are the same or react the same to medications. The neurologist may need to try several different drugs in different combinations before he finds the right "cocktail." And then, as the dementia progresses, the way the drugs work may change and the neurologist may again have to experiment and adjust or even change that cocktail altogether. As part of the care team, professionals can reassure family members that such continual experimenting is actually good medicine.

Balancing Medications

PD Drugs

Motor symptoms are treated with medications like Sinemet (carbidopa/levodopa). They tend to work well--until the Lewy bodies begin to migrate out of the midbrain and into areas controlling cognition and dementia symptoms begin to appear.

PD meds tend to make dementia symptoms worse or cause symptoms when none were previously present. Therefore, at the first sign of dementia, a Lewy-savvy neurologist will usually cut back on the PD medications. This often works and for a while the cognition issues will disappear. However, this does not curb any cognitive decline that is being caused by the Lewy bodies.

Eventually, the neurologist will likely add one of the ChEIs. Then there may be another balance issue. While the dementia drug may improve cognition and decrease hallucinations, it may also cause parkinsonism, decreasing motor function even more. Doctor, family and patient may have to choose between better mobility and better cognition--or hopefully, find some acceptable balance between the two.

When Mom started showing dementia symptoms, her neurologist cut back on her Sinemet. She is able to think better but now she has to use a walker. Even so, we both agreed that if we had to choose, we'd take awareness over movement. - Marion Peterson

Most family caregivers report that they would choose better cognition even when the loss of their patient's mobility increases their workload.

Remember how I said that David started having tremors. Well, his doctor changed him from Aricept to Exelon to Razadyne, trying to find the best medication. Razadyne seemed to work the best but he still has a small tremor. His neurologist tried giving him a small dose of PD meds. That stopped the tremors but David went back to having hallucinations! His doctor is still trying to find the right drug cocktail for him. - Marie Newman

DLB families like the Newmans face similar choices to that of PDD families although their focus is only on balancing cognition medications and the possible side effect of "parkinsonism."

Antipsychotics

The antipsychotic drugs designed to treat hallucinations, delusions and other psychotic symptoms are generally contraindicated for anyone living with LBD although even Lewy-savvy doctors may prescribe some of the milder ones off-label and in small doses with careful monitoring to help manage the LBD-related behavioral and psychotic symptoms that have not responded to other treatment. See Chapter 25, Behavior Management.

13. Non-Drug Therapy

exercise: Activity requiring physical effort.

healthy diet: A diet that includes those nutrients needed to maintain health, energy and happiness.

mental stimulation: Anything that stimulates the brain and increases its mental reserves.

socialization: Interacting with other people.

***

Experts worldwide agree that certain non-drug options are very helpful at decreasing the risk of dementia. Once there are symptoms, that changes and very little can stop the disease's progress. These measures will help a person living with LBD to have fewer symptoms and a better quality of life but they probably won't live any longer.

Socialization

Being around people may not slow dementia but isolation is quite likely to speed it up! Humans are "herd animals." We do best when we are around other people. However, that can be difficult as failing mental and physical abilities make interacting with others more difficult. Socialization is beginning to be recognized as every bit as important as exercise for keeping dementia at bay and managing its symptoms.[18]

> *Action:* Bring the socialization to the person. If the person lives at home, encourage the care partner to invite one, or no more than two, friends to visit for an hour or so. If they live in a care center, encourage in-house one-on-one friendships and encourage visitors to come one or two at a time. Groups are too stressful and decrease a person's ability to socialize.

Mental Stimulation

As with socialization, mental stimulation isn't likely to slow down the progress of the disease once it is present. But it may help a person stay sharp for a longer period of time. It definitely adds quality to one's life. Because memory lasts longer for a person living with LBD than it does for someone with Alzheimer's, they may still be able to learn for quite a while after cognitive symptoms appear. It will take longer and many more repetitions than it did before but it can happen.[19]

Any kind of brain stimulation is good: puzzles, reading a book, writing, memory games, having a hobby that keeps you busy. The best kind of mental stimulation is where the patient learns something new and different. People—including the elderly and especially those with dementia—need challenges to keep their minds keen. How well one does on the task isn't important; what is important is that being challenged keeps the brain stimulated. Stimulation oxygenates the brain and keeps it functioning at an optimum level.

With dementia, challenge remains important but it manifests differently. For the LBD patient, maintaining a semblance of normalcy is the challenge. A good attitude helps. If you focus more on the fun of the challenge than on the results, the patient will usually reflect this and become less discouraged. With dementia, it is the journey, not the destination that counts.

With someone whose dementia is more apparent, activities like scrapbooking[20] can be very helpful, especially if you incorporate old photos or the patient's stories of their past life, family, etc. The work is active; the photos and mementos stimulate memory and doing it with someone else provides social interaction.

Mom started scrapbooking years ago. At first she had to make them "just so." Now we have fun sitting together and reading her old scrapbooks, talking about the people in the pictures and what was happening. - Marion Peterson

Mrs. Peterson made scrapbooking a challenge. Now, these same books provide a vehicle for Mrs. Peterson to exercise her memory as she and Marion review the books. Looking at them together is also a social time—something that happens less often as the communication skills decrease.

Action: Adjust mental challenges to abilities so that they neither bore nor overburden. Adapt old hobbies so that they can still be enjoyed and find new ways, such as reminiscing, to continue to stimulate the mental processes.

Exercise

It has long been believed that exercise was a better treatment for dementia than any drug. This may not be quite true. While there is strong evidence that life-long exercise can reduce a person's risk of dementia by as much as a whopping 88%, the latest research didn't find that it slowed down dementia once there are symptoms.[21]

Nevertheless, exercise remains important. Even though cognitive advantages may be limited, physical fitness makes self-care easier which in turn improves self-esteem and decreases the likelihood of dementia-related behaviors. It can decrease anxiety, which will also decrease those behaviors. It improves cardiovascular and metabolic health, both of which help a person make better use of what brain power is still available.

A regular regimen of exercise several times a week remains best but any is better than none. Chair exercises are helpful when a person's mobility is limited. Doing exercises in a group adds to the effectiveness because of the added social interaction.

David and I have been square dancers for a long time and we still go. It's hard for David sometimes when he forgets something he's known for years but we aren't quitting. This kind of exercise is just too important! - Marie Newman

Square dancing is great group exercise for patients with mild LBD. There's usually someone to pull them through the moves they forget. There's sociability and there is lots of repetition. And don't discount the togetherness, something that often becomes scarce for couples when LBD appears.

Peter and I do exercises every morning. I get my exercise exercising him! I wish he could go to the group and do chair exercises the way

Mrs. Peterson and Mrs. Ashton do but he just isn't able to do that anymore. We do them right in his bed, before he gets up in the morning. Sometimes, he can do a lot of them. Sometimes, I'm doing most of the work, pushing his legs and arms around so they get some movement. - Jenny Ellis

When Mrs. Ellis moves her husband's limbs back and forth, this is "passive exercise." It is not as good for a person as moving one's muscle personally but it is better than no exercise at all.

The exercise should be challenging but not overwhelming and thus, discouraging. Variety is also important but as dementia progresses, this becomes less so. The challenge changes to be simply being able to do anything at all.

> *Action:* Maintaining an exercise program for a person whose mental abilities continue to degenerate over time and whose apathy may limit cooperation can be a challenge for family care partner and care staff. Make exercise fun by choosing things the patient likes to do and doing them with the patient. The square dancing that the Newmans do is a good example.

Combining Skills

Activities that combine the use of more than one skill are best. Perhaps that is why socialization is so good. It usually requires a variety of skills, depending on how it is being done. An activity such as dancing, for example, can include learning new steps, relate to others and physical exercise. This is much more than doing a word puzzle, a sit-down visit or even a solitary walk around the block.

Healthy Diet

No specific foods have been firmly identified for cognition preservation. However, there have been many studies that showed support for certain kinds of food decreasing the risk of dementia, including those in the Mediterranean diet:[22] This diet is high in fish, legumes, fruit, vegetables and olive oil and low in dairy foods, red meat and eggs.

Hilda was a good cook but she stopped when she started burning stuff in the frying pan. Of course, she blamed the pan! When I took over the cooking, I did some research about what helped dementia and what didn't. We started eating more fish and more vegetables. Who knows—maybe that's why Hilda's symptoms are still mild—that and all the exercising we do. - Barney Darnell

Barney could be right. Their proactive approach could very well be helping to limit Hilda's LBD symptoms. Good diet and adequate exercise are two of the ways that one can maintain a certain amount of control over an uncontrollable and unpredictable disease like LBD.

Alcohol And Coffee

While both alcohol and coffee have been shown to be helpful in lowering the risk of dementia, this is another one that changes with the advent of dementia symptoms, especially if LBD is involved. Alcohol often conflicts with cognition and other medications. Coffee is a mild diuretic and when it becomes difficult to get liquids down, it is not as good as water or juice for maintaining good fluid balance.

Other Symptoms

Although the cognitive dysfunctions of dementia are the most well-known LBD symptoms, or at least the ones the disease is named for, there are many more.

- Drug sensitivity
- Fluctuating cognition
- Perceptual issues such as hallucinations
- Sleep disorders, such as Active Dreams
- Parkinsonism, or motor symptoms
- Autonomic System dysfunctions such as low blood pressure on rising.
- Mood disorders such as apathy

These issues combined with the previously mentioned cognitive deficits lead to a variety of dementia-related behaviors which are often the most difficult part of this disease to handle.

14. Fluctuating Cognition

fluctuating cognition: A defining LBD symptom where cognition fluctuates up and down instead of declining regularly.

Good Times: When a patient is more alert and aware.

Bad Times: When a patient is more confused.

Showtime: When a patient acts "normal" for a limited time in the presence of someone other than their caregiver.

***

Mrs. Ashton has Alzheimer's. Her cognitive abilities have declined gradually from the start of her disease to the present. Mrs. Peterson's cognitive abilities fluctuate from month to month and even minute to minute, as her LBD progresses.

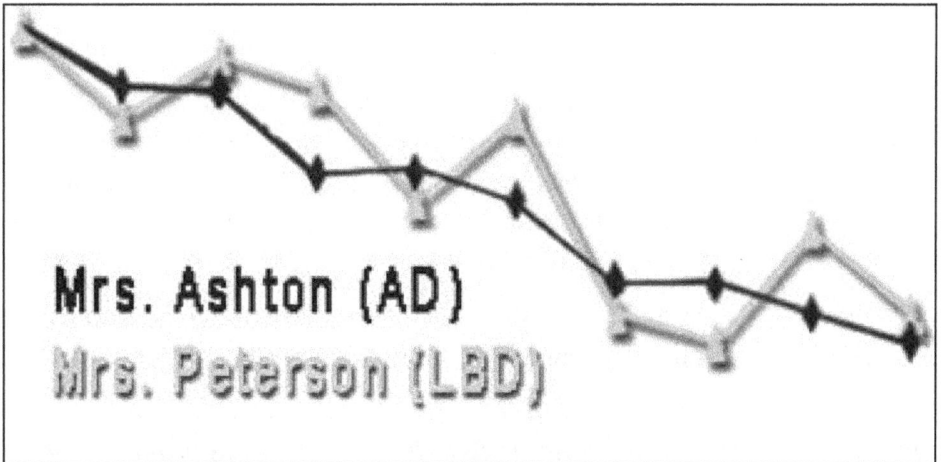

Mrs. Ashton (AD)
Mrs. Peterson (LBD)

This simulated chart shows the decline of general cognitive functioning for Mrs. Ashton and Mrs. Peterson over a ten month period. Notice that while the cognitive functioning of both women has declined an equal amount, there are differences: Mrs. Ashton's path is a gradual downward slide. Mrs. Peterson's is more of a roller coaster ride, with the amount of cognition rising on occasion and at other times plunging to great depths.

The improved cognition seldom lasts and the patient seldom recovers fully from the plunges. Although these downward dips in cognition are a normal part of the progression of the disease, they can also follow a period of illness or an injury and are often medication related. Although the patient's cognitive ability may improve at times, it will seldom reach the level that it was prior to the illness or injury.

My grandmother thought I was my mom the last time I visited and this time, she didn't know me at all. I'm not sure why I keep coming! Well, she does act like she enjoys having me visit even when she doesn't know who I am. I see other changes too. She's beginning to have trouble dressing and undressing and she doesn't seem to care what she says anymore. - Janice Ashton

From one visit to the next, Janice can see that her grandmother's memory is worse as are her inhibitions. Even her ability to perform her activities of daily living without supervision is decreasing. Her decline has been gradual, a slide down with few if any recoveries.

This is not true for Mrs. Peterson. Marion brought her grown son to the group and he shared his observations about his grandmother.

I visit Grandma every week and I never know how I'll find her. Sometimes, she remembers me and sometimes she doesn't. Sometimes, she can feed herself and sometimes she can't. Sometimes we can have a reasonable conversation and sometimes, well, sometimes Grandma acts scared of me, or angry—or just ignores me. It's so sad. - Jonathan

Mrs. Peterson's cognitive abilities vary from visit to visit, improving and decreasing erratically. However, there are some patterns.

Mom is usually better, a little more aware and a little more able to perform her ADLs when Jonathan is visiting. Mom might have several days in a row where she feels more normal even when he isn't here but it never lasts. She always has a 'bad spell' again. - Marion

Yes, and I know her condition is worse than it was this time last year, or even last month. - Jonathan

Looking back over the last year of ups and downs, Jonathan can see that his grandmother's cognition has decreased significantly. His grandmother will rally and appear better for a while but then her abilities decrease and she can do even less than before. The worst decline came after a bout of severe colitis. When she recovered, her best periods of awareness were not as clear as her "norm" had been before her illness.

It was a much quicker decline for Peter. He and I were doing just fine in the assisted living wing before he fell. Peter had some mild dementia symptoms but it didn't interfere with our active life. We traveled, had friends in for visits and were Foster Grandparents. That all changed when he fell and broke his hip. He's not the same anymore. - Jenny Ellis

Mr. Ellis went from mild to advanced LBD after his fall and the surgery for his broken hip. His awareness plunged and other LBD symptoms, such as hallucinations increased. He still has flashes of awareness but they seldom last long and he almost never talks now.

When the group talks about their loved one's fluctuations, they call them "the Good Times," "the Bad Times," and "the Showtimes."

The Good Times

These are the norms at first: an alert, aware person with periods of occasional confusion. The disease starts very gradually, with short little incidents of confusion and dementia-related behavior. At that point families seldom consider dementia. Grandma acts a bit odd now and then. However, most of the time she is as alert and aware as she always was, so they don't worry about it. Eventually the good times become less frequent although they never disappear entirely.

The presence of these good times is one of the big differences between Alzheimer's and LBD. Mrs. Ashton goes along in a gathering fog, gradually becoming less and less aware of her effect on others. Mrs. Peterson has windows of awareness, where she can relate with family and where she has a better picture of what her life is like. Although this ability can be both positive and negative, family caregivers tend to value highly these special times.

Lynn Davis wrote the following poem about her husband. It describes a "good time" that they experienced and how fleeting it was.

An Old Flame

Yesterday I had a chance encounter with an old flame.

He was every bit as charming as I remember.

I was so glad to see him. We had dinner together

And talked about everything and nothing at all.

It made me feel young again and yes, I even flirted a little.

It was just so nice to spend an evening being "normal".

I don't recall exactly when he left.

I just looked up and John was gone

and Lewy had returned.

The Bad Times

Gradually, the confusion and dementia-related behavior, the "bad times," become the norm, with periods of less confusion showing up occasionally, as they did for Lynn and her husband. However, this is a degenerative disease. Even when the good times do appear, the level of functioning will not be as high as it used to be and these special times won't last as long as they did previously.

Peter is confused most of the time now—his day is made up mostly of "bad times." However, he still has windows of awareness and I've learned to save my questions and news for those times. - Jenny Ellis.

Mr. Ellis tends to be more alert when he is most rested, likely in the morning or after a nap. Staff has also learned to arrange his schedule to take advantage of his windows of awareness, although they know they can't count on them appearing on a regular basis.

Sometimes Mrs. Peterson can talk as plain as I can. At others, she either won't say anything or she just mumbles. I sometimes think she's just lazy and doesn't want to bother. - Beverly - care staff.

Mrs. Peterson isn't lazy and she isn't faking or ignoring Beverly. She has no control over her cognitive level from one moment to the next.

Action: Use patience and acceptance. Being irritable will only make Mrs. Peterson's symptoms worse. As much as possible, Beverly should schedule her activities such as bathing during times when she is most alert and able to participate.

The Showtimes

When a patient acts "normal" for a limited time in the presence of someone other than their caregiver, we call this Showtime. Most of us have an ingrained impulse to show our best side to those we deem important. For the LBD patient, that includes people like the doctor and visiting family members. People with a healthy brain can choose to do this or not. Without impulse control, a LBD patient can't choose. They will go with that first impulse.

Jake has become so combative that sometimes I can't handle him alone. I called my step-sons and told them Jake needed to move to some place like Anytown where he'd be safer. His oldest, Harold, came out for a couple of days to see what I was talking about. And wouldn't you know it, the whole time he was here, Jake was on Showtime! Harold even suggested that maybe I had the problem! - Norma Dupree

Thanks to Showtime, Harold saw his father acting a bit absent minded and slower, not much different than last time he saw him. Harold knew his father had bad dreams and sometime he saw things but he didn't see this as a reason to place their father in an institution. Thus, he suspected his youngish step-mother of feeling tied down and wanting out.

Luckily, Harold went with the Duprees to visit Jake's physician, a Lewy-savvy man. He explained about the normal fluctuations that anyone with LBD will experience and about Showtime. Jake is now waiting for a room to come available in the Anytown dementia wing.

Showtime can also be a challenge for the physician whose patient acts out at home but appears perfectly normal during office visits. Since this is an illness treated symptom by symptom, the best way for the physician to know what to prescribe is by observing the patient and their behavior.

Marion laughs when she tells about Mrs. Peterson's Showtime:

As soon as we enter the doctor's office, Mom straightens up and talks better than she ever does at home. Then when we leave she slumps again and quits talking. But it's really hard on Mom. She sleeps most of the next day. - Marion Peterson

It isn't only the dementia that improves. Mrs. Peterson, who has had PD for years, also can have better motor and language skills for a short time. Mrs. Peterson's sleeping the next day is understandable.

Showtime is physically and mentally taxing. It can take several days to recover.

Treatment

There is no specific treatment for fluctuating cognition. Rather, it is a learning process, where the care partner and staff learn when best to work with the patient and what to expect.

- *Cognition drugs.* These drugs may help with all LBD symptoms including fluctuating cognition.
- *Non-drug therapy.* Although nothing is going to stop the progression to more "bad times," anything that adds comfort and decreases stress is going to make them less troublesome. Our books, Managing Cognitive Issues and Responsive Dementia Care, both offer many specific suggestions.
- *Documentation.* A daily record of a patient's behaviors and fluctuations over time can help the physician and non-resident relatives understand a patient's actual needs. Some care partners have even used video cameras or their phone videos to more eloquently document behavior changes.

15. Parkinsonism

acetylcholine: A neurotransmitter in the brain cortex that facilitates cognition.

dopamine: A neurotransmitter in the midbrain that facilitates mobility.

parkinsonism: A collective name for motor and mobility symptoms such as those that show up in Parkinson's but also in other diseases including DLB.

***

Motor symptoms are usually the first noticeable symptoms to show up with Parkinson's (PD). These continue on into Parkinson's with dementia (PDD), getting worse as the disease progresses. Although they tend to show up much later with dementia with Lewy bodies (DLB) and seldom get as severe, parkinsonism is almost always present. And like PD's motor symptoms, they will likely last and get worse as the disease progresses.

Mom's first symptoms were barely noticeable. She complained about "shaking inside" but I couldn't see a tremor. And she got a lot slower but I thought that was just age, until she started shuffling. It was when she fell because her balance was so poor that we knew she was truly losing her mobility. That's when the doctor diagnosed her with Parkinson's. By then, her "inside tremor" was real, most obvious when she wasn't using her hands. - Marion Peterson

With PD, a person's first symptoms will usually be muscle related. Mrs. Peterson's feeling of shaking inside is from tremors too subtle to see. Aching, tingling and burning may accompany these invisible symptoms. Muscle stiffness and rigidity, slow movements, balance problems, shuffling gait, tremors, loss of dexterity, stooped posture, blank facial expression and small handwriting all become that person's new way of life. It can be decades before a diagnosis of PDD occurs. Mrs. Peterson can expect her motor symptoms to last, becoming even worse as the disease progresses.

People living with DLB may also have motor symptoms but they start later. In fact, when these symptoms start is the main way to tell which kind of LBD a person has: PDD or DLB. If motor symptoms come first, it is called PDD. That's the way it was for Mrs. Peterson. She had the shuffling gait, the stooped posture and other Parkinson's symptoms long before any dementia symptoms were evident.

If the motor symptoms don't show up until well after cognitive symptoms are present, the disease is called DLB. That's the way it was for David Newman. However, Lewy bodies may not be the cause of these early mobility issues.

David didn't have any motor problems until his doctor put him on a dementia medication. Then he developed a tremor and even worse, his arms began to contract and he could hardly move them. The doctor changed David's medication and the tremor stopped. - Marie Newman

Motor dysfunctions that appear after the advent of dementia may be due to drugs the patient is taking for dementia. PD meds and dementia meds require balancing because each may decrease the effectiveness of the other. As with everything else about Lewy body disease, this varies with each individual. Someone else may have been able to tolerate the new drugs well...or they might have responded even more drastically.

David doesn't have tremors anymore but now, he's having trouble swallowing and his balance is poor. He doesn't show his emotions like he used to either. I know he still feels them but his face doesn't seem to be able to move enough to express them. The doctor says she doesn't believe these symptoms are drug related this time. - Marie Newman

Even though the change of medication stopped David's tremors initially, parkinsonism of some sort is likely to reappear as his disease advances. As his doctor said, these later symptoms are more likely to be Lewy body related rather than drug related.

Unexplained rigidity, falls and problems with hand use are all common DLB motor symptoms. Facial muscles and throat muscles often become impaired, causing blank expressions and swallowing difficulties like David's. However, DLB care partners report that their loved one's mobility symptoms are seldom as severe as those of people living with PDD. Even so, as the disease advances a walker may be needed or occasionally, even a wheelchair.

Treatment

Since the neurotransmitters, dopamine and acetylcholine, require a balance of strengths for both to function well, increasing one tends to interfere with the function of the other. Parkinson's drugs[23] work to improve the action of dopamine, which facilitates mobility.

- Some, such as Levodopa, increase dopamine levels in the brain.
- Others, such as Requip (ropinirole), mimic dopamine.
- Still others, such as Cogentin (benzotropine mesylate), act as anticholinergics, which increases dopamine ratio compared to acetylcholine.

All tend to work well until the onset of cognitive issues. Then any of these drugs can make cognition even worse, although the anticholinergics are the most likely to do so.

Conversely, the cognition drugs can increase parkinsonism symptoms. Treatment of these symptoms in PDD usually starts with a decrease of Parkinson's drugs and continues via trial and error until the physician finds the best balance of drugs for both mobility and cognition. In DLB, treatment for parkinsonism symptoms likely consists of an addition of PD drugs with careful monitoring followed by trial and error testing until the right combination is found.

Since these diseases are degenerative however, conditions will continue to change and it is always important to remember that what works today may not work as well or even at all tomorrow.

16. Drug Sensitivity

Anti-anxiety drugs: (aka: tranquilizers): Drugs used to treat anxiety and agitation and as a muscle relaxant.

Anticholinergic drug: (anti-koh-luh-nur-jik) One that impairs or weakens acetylcholine. Includes muscle relaxants, anti-anxiety drugs, sedatives and antipsychotics. Most are Lewy-sensitive.

Anti-dopaminergic drug: (anti-doh-puh-mi-nur-jik) One that impairs or weakens dopamine. Includes most dementia drugs.

Antipsychotics: (aka: neuroleptics) Drugs approved for treating psychotic symptoms in psychiatric diseases such as schizophrenia and often used "off label" with dementia.

black box warning: FDA required warning on all antipsychotic product packaging[24] that the use of antipsychotics in the elderly is linked to increased risk of serious illness and death.

drug sensitivity: The reaction to a normal dose as though it were an overdose. Varies greatly with each individual and each drug.

Lewy sensitive drug: A drug known to trigger drug sensitivity in some people living with LBD. Includes most antipsychotics, anti-anxiety drugs, sedatives and anticholinergics.

Lewy-sensitivity: Drug sensitivity brought on by the interaction of the drug and LBD:

paradoxical reaction: A reaction opposite to that expected, usually resulting in an increase rather than decrease of the treated symptom.

sedatives: Drugs used as sleeping aids and to treat anxiety.

***

Lewy-sensitivity, or drug sensitivity connected to Lewy bodies, occurs when the Lewy bodies have already compromised and weakened a drug's target. This is the case with *anticholinergics*, drugs that target *acetylcholine*. As Lewy bodies spread out in the cognitive areas of the brain, they begin to come into contact with this neurotransmitter. Then when an anticholinergic drug is taken the person gets a double hit, once from the Lewy bodies and once from the drug, greatly increasing the chances of drug sensitivity.

Like most LBD symptoms drug sensitivity is very individual, in that no two people react the same way. One person can have a very severe reaction to a drug and the next person, with equally advanced dementia, may not react at all. For the patient, family and doctor, the use of these drugs can become a trial and error situation. The Lewy-savvy doctor starts out very low, increases slowly, monitors carefully and stops the drug at any sign of sensitivity.

A person may suddenly become sensitive to a drug after being able to take it without a problem for years. That's because their Lewy bodies have migrated into the cognitive areas of their brain where acetylcholine is more common. They will probably begin to show other signs of this too, such as hallucinations or even delusions.

My sister had hallucinations and delusions after taking her pain medication but not at any other time. - Ellen

Miss Cleary's symptoms are likely evidence of a beginning drug sensitivity related to her Parkinson's disease. She and Ellen can also use it as a warning that other drug sensitivities and cognitive symptoms are likely to show up in the near future.

The hospice nurse cut the dose in half but the hallucinations still showed up. So then she cut that in half and the hallucinations didn't come back. I wondered if that small a dose would even do her any good but it did. - Ellen

The sensitivity that made the drugs strong enough to cause the unwanted side-effects also made it strong enough for very little to do its intended job. This can often be the case with Lewy-sensitivity. The doctor may try cutting the dose before changing the medication.

Although opiates can be Lewy-sensitive, behavior management drugs are the greatest culprits. Most are anticholinergics in addition to their intended action, which can also be less than supportive of the Lewy body damaged brain. For example, sedatives slow down the central nervous system already compromised by Lewy bodies. Side effects include heavy sedation, confusion, increased dementia symptoms and sometimes, an adverse reaction--the increase of the symptom the drug was supposed to treat.

Drugs At Highest Risk For Lewy-Sensitivity

Inhaled anesthetics. Inhaled anesthetics act to slow down the central nervous system during surgery. These drugs should be used with extreme care with all elderly people. Their nervous systems are already compromised by age. Add LBD, which also compromises the nervous system and these drugs become much more risky. They should be avoided or used with an understanding of likely results.

We were living in the Anytown assisted living wing when Peter fell. Before that, he would have spells of confusion, occasional mild hallucinations and active dreams but on the whole he was able to communicate and enjoy life. After the surgery to repair his broken hip his confusion got a lot worse. Then he became combative and they told me he'd have to move to the dementia wing where there was more supervision and assistance. That's where he is now. - Jenny Ellis

Caregiver sites abound with stories of loved ones who had surgery followed by major, often permanent cognitive losses similar to those displayed by Mr. Ellis.

Scientific papers are beginning to support this finding. It can cause a quandary for the physician and family of a LBD patient who needs surgery. Do they go ahead with the surgery, knowing that it may cause a severe decrease in cognition? If it is a matter of relieving major pain, they may. But if the surgery is to extend life, like heart repair, the family may choose to let the patient live as they are. This is an individual choice; the decision will vary with the problem and the people involved. Mr. Ellis had been in great pain after the fall. Both he and his wife wanted the surgery even though they knew the risks.

These older and stronger drugs should be avoided altogether. In most cases there are newer, gentler drugs that can be used instead.

First generation antidepressants. Strong sedatives and strong anticholinergics, these drugs are seldom used anymore because there are newer, safer choices. Examples: amitriptyline (Elivil), methyldopa (Aldomet), phenelzine (Nardil) and tranylcypromine (Parnate). While not in the above class, Paxil (paroxentine) is a SSRI antidepressant with greater anticholinergic action than others in its class.

Traditional antipsychotics: These drugs are a) not FDA approved for use with dementia, b) carry a black-box warning that they are especially risky for dementia patients and c) are usually quite strong. The only one still in regular use is Haldol (haloperidol). It is sometimes used as an inexpensive drug in hospital emergency rooms and hospice services to calm difficult patients. Symptoms can be severe and sometimes even permanent. They include confusion, heavy sedation, parkinsonism and in rare cases, neuroleptic malignant syndrome (fever, rigidity, possible kidney failure).

When I tried to explain to Jake that he needed more help than I could give at home, he became combative. He insisted that I didn't love him anymore and that I just wanted to get rid of him. I tried to calm him down but finally I just had to call 911. The paramedics took Jake to the local emergency room where the staff treated him traditionally with Haldol. I tried to tell them that he shouldn't have it but the nurse told me not to worry, that this is what they always did and it wouldn't cause any problem. Well, Jake's arms are still rigid and barely move because of that one shot. - Norma Dupree

Soon after this, Norma obtained an LBDA Medical Alert wallet card[25]. This card lists those medications that may cause problems for LBD patients. Norma keeps it with her to give to ER staff or other medical personnel who may not be familiar with her husband's history. She also made sure that Haldol was listed as an allergy on his medical records.

Drugs At High Risk For Lewy-Sensitivity

While still strongly anticholinergic, the following drugs were once thought to be less immediately damaging for people with other kinds of dementia such as Alzheimers. That has changed in the last few years. These drugs are not recommended for use by anyone with any kind of dementia and should be avoided or used with extreme caution and close monitoring.

Benzodiazepines. Sedative drugs with anticholinergic properties used to treat anxiety, insomnia and allergies. Examples: clorazepate (Tranxene), diazepam (Valium) and alprazolam (Xanax). Heavy sedation is a common symptom. Other symptoms include parkinsonism, confusion and paradoxical reactions all of which can be very long-lasting and possibly permanent.

Sleeping aids. Sedative drugs with anticholinergic properties used as sleep aids. Examples: zolpidem (Ambien), eszopiclone (Lunesta) or zaleplon (Sonata). Symptoms include heavy sedation, parkinsonism and confusion.

Drugs At Milder Risk For Lewy-Sensitivity

The following drugs can still cause serious Lewy-sensitive reactions in some people. They should be used with caution and in the smallest workable dose, monitored carefully and stopped at the first sign of sensitivity.

Atypical antipsychotics.[26] These second generation antipsychotics are still not approved for use with dementia patients and also carry the black box warning. However, this threat of future problems has not been enough to stop their often successful use for immediate treatment. This isn't as negative as it sounds. When care partners and doctors have to choose between a longer but unhappy life and a shorter, more comfortable life for the patient, they often find this an easy choice, especially when nothing else has worked. Ex: Seroquel (quetiapine), Risperdal (risperidone) Abilify (aripiprazole).

Jake's doctor prescribed Seroquel to curb his combativeness. It worked and he did settle down and go to sleep. But then, he had such bad dreams that he kept me awake all night. - Norma Dupree

Mom takes Seroquel and she hasn't had any problems at all. - Marion Peterson

Other caregivers have reported similar good and bad results with this and other atypicals. This variety of results underlines the diversity of this disease. It is different with every patient and every patient will respond differently to medication.

SSRI antidepressants. The family of selective serotonin reuptake inhibitors (SSRIs)[27] may be prescribed for depression and even anxiety but with limited success. They are more effective for the depressed care partner. Ex: Zoloft (sertraline), Prozac (fluoxetine), Celexa (citalopram). The exception is Paxil (paroxetine) which is a stronger anticholinergic than its sister drugs and *should be avoided*. Its use is correlated with high dementia risk later in life.

Other antidepressants. Wellbutrin (bupropion) and Remeron (mirtazapine) are milder drugs often prescribed for depression with LBD.

Opiates and other prescription pain drugs. Caregivers also repeatedly report that their loved ones are overly sensitive to opiates like morphine and Demerol or other strong analgesics, expressing hallucinations, delusions and other dementia-related behaviors with normal doses. This can be true, not only for LBD but for PD as well.

My sister's hallucinations actually showed up first when she was hospitalized for cancer treatment and given some very strong pain medications. She also started believing that the staff was plotting against her. Even after she left the hospital and was no longer taking the medication, she continued to believe her danger was real and was terrified at the thought of going into the hospital again. However, she only hallucinated or had more delusions at home when the hospice nurse medicated her for pain. - Ellen

Miss Cleary's response to pain drugs is common for someone with advanced PD. The persistence of her delusional fear is classic for LBD-related delusions. They show that the Lewy bodies have begun to invade the thinking areas of her brain. However, the fact that neither they nor the hallucinations show up without a drug trigger suggests that the Lewy bodies haven't spread very far.

Over-the-counter medications. Many sleep or allergy aids contain Benadryl (diphenhydramine) or other antihistamines. These drugs have an anticholinergic effect that can cause extreme side effects in LBD patients, similar to those of antipsychotics or tranquilizers. For the same reason, they may also interfere with the effectiveness of cognition medications. However, these non-prescription drugs tend to be milder and don't stay in the body as long and so the sensitivity is usually less intense.

Hilda has seasonal allergies and has always used antihistamines with good results. But that changed after she started taking cognition meds.

She got really confused and it lasted for several hours. Then she was fine again but I didn't give her any more antihistamines! - Barney Darnell

Unlike tranquilizers, which can cause very long lasting, possibly permanent confusion, the effect of Hilda's antihistamines was temporary and wore off when the medication left her body.

Drug Overuse

The inappropriate use of antipsychotics, anti-anxiety drugs, opiates and sedatives is most likely to occur in care facilities. They are in the business to make a profit. They may also want to provide good service but the bottom line is that if they don't make a profit they will cease to exist.

I know the staff here really wants to help Mom but she is only one of the far too many residents assigned to one caregiver. That means that she gets ignored a lot. Thank goodness, I'm there to take up a lot of the slack for her but I've noticed that other less fortunate residents who fuss get medicated fairly quickly. – Marion Peterson

Marion's concern about staff size is valid. Staff salaries are a facilities largest expense. Cutting staff size is therefore the quickest way to economize. For years behavior management drugs such as those in the above categories including even the most risky, have been used to keep patients quiet and agreeable so that care staff can carry bigger patient loads.

In 2012, the federal government began a program aimed at drastically reducing the use of antipsychotic drugs in nursing homes. Since then, the use of these drugs has decreased but not enough. The problem remains. A 2018 survey showed that drugs were still being used simply to make patients easier to handle.[28]

I've had directives put into Mom's chart that due to her sensitivities, she isn't to be given any drug without my permission. So far, I haven't had a problem but I've talked to other care partners with family in other facilities where their directives were actually ignored. - Marion Peterson

Marion's observation about directives is true. That 2018 survey showed that drugs were given without consent. Often, the facility will describe the event as a crisis where they had to act quickly. That events are regularly allowed to escalate to that level shows a lack of training about LBD care and likely, too few staff.

PD and Dementia Drugs

Both PD and dementia drugs can interfere with the action of other drugs given for a Lewy body disease. Acetylcholine, which facilitates cognition and dopamine, which facilitates mobility, function in a ratio relationship. That is, when one is higher than normal it decreases the effect of the other. Likewise, when one is lower it increases the effect of the other.

Some PD drugs. These drugs increase mobility by decreasing acetylcholine's action instead of increasing that of dopamine to get better mobility. This works well until the Lewy bodies get into the cognitive areas of the brain. When cognitive symptoms first appear with PD, the doctor will usually decrease the PD meds and/or change them to drugs with less of an anticholinergic action. Example: Symmetrel (amantadine), Artane (trihexyphenidyl), Cogentin (benztropine mesylate).

Dementia drugs. Aricept (donepezil), Exelon (rivastigmine) and Razadyne (galantamine) increase cognition by acting to increase acetylcholine, thus decreasing the effect of dopamine and causing the possibility of parkinsonism symptoms to occur.

17. Visual Symptoms

Capgras syndrome: Viewing the care partner as a look-alike imposter.

depth perception: The ability to judge the distance between themselves and others.

hand-eye coordination: The ability to coordinate vision with hand movements.

illusions: Misidentifying something that is there.

visual hallucinations: Seeing something that isn't really there. A defining LBD symptom.

***

The symptoms in this chapter often occur well before any cognitive symptoms. The early appearance of visual hallucinations is a defining LBD symptom, one that helps the physician choose a LBD diagnosis rather than one for Alzheimer's.

Hallucinations

Visual hallucinations, or seeing something that isn't there, can appear early in the progress of the disease and may be the first recognizable symptom of LBD. Visual hallucinations may be caused by a person's overactive visual cortex, resulting in images being generated in the brain of things that aren't actually there. People living with PD often experience hallucinations that they know are not real. With intact thinking abilities, they can understand and accept that these visions are a part of their illness. However, as their illness progresses and thinking abilities decline, they will begin to believe their hallucinations are real.

Most hallucinations are benign and may bother the care partner more than they do the patient. While they may not be scary, these false visions are usually quite realistic and detailed. They can reoccur, becoming dramas that may last over time.[29]

Jake often sees children coming out from behind the TV set. At first that really bothered me but I realized that they didn't bother him. In fact he liked the company. So now I just smile and nod. - Norma Dupree

Jake's hallucinations were benign; they bothered him less than they did Norma. She did the right thing to relax and let it go

Mom used to know when her hallucinations weren't real. She'd tell me that she saw kids in the room and I'd tell her I didn't see any and she'd shrug and nod. She knew that hallucinations were PD symptoms too. But now, she gets upset if I don't agree with her. - Marion Peterson

Mrs. Peterson's PD has progressed into PDD. She is no longer able to use her thinking abilities to accept what she sees as a symptom of her illness. They have become real to her and she is hurt when her daughter challenges her.

> **Action:** Once a person can't tell that they are having hallucinations, don't try to change their reality. You will only make things worse. As long as they aren't bothering the patient, let them be and encourage care partners to do so also. If they want validation from you give it. You don't have to "see" what they see but you do have to accept that they do and "play along." "I know you see it but I don't," probably won't work once a person's thinking abilities fade. The person will feel discounted.

None of the above patients were frightened by their hallucinations. However, this is not always the case.

Peter was a soldier in Viet Nam and now he thinks that he's back there. He sees the jungle and other stuff that he's never wanted to talk about. He still doesn't talk about it but he cringes and shudders and I know he's reliving those awful times. - Jenny Ellis

These frightening hallucinations are probably linked to some PTSD, driven by bad dreams about his war years, delusions and general confusion.

> **Action:** With bothersome hallucinations, join their reality and move the action in a way that will improve the situation. For example, Norma might usher Jake's "children" out the door or Jenny might tell her husband that she saw the enemy soldiers leave.

Illusions

Unlike hallucinations where the patient sees something that isn't there at all, illusions are seeing something that is there but seeing it incorrectly. It's more of a thinking error, a faulty identification of something perceived. For instance, a patient may see a small animal instead of a shoe box.

We traveled a lot before Peter fell. Once, when we were seated near the back of the plane, Peter nudged me, pointed forward and whispered to me. He wanted to know if I saw a fire up there. I looked and all I could see was a flickering TV screen. I told him that and he didn't act worried anymore. - Jenny Ellis

Mr. Ellis was seeing an illusion but because his thinking abilities were still fairly intact, he could accept his wife's explanation. He might even have been able to readjust his perceptions so that he actually saw the TV instead of the fire.

Mom has a 'pet,' a little dog she keeps seeing, especially if there's something like a box or a shoe on the floor. She says it keeps her company. - Marion Peterson

Mrs. Peterson isn't frightened of her "pet" and may or may not believe it is really there. Illusions are seldom as troubling or as real as hallucinations can become.

Capgras Syndrome

These are a special kind of delusion, where a person sees a loved one as an impostor who looks like their loved one but isn't.[30] They have been called "the illusion of doubles" and defined as "an interpretative illusion, rather than misperception of external stimuli." or more simply put, "seeing the person correctly but being delusional about who they are." However you want to define them, their saving grace is that they only occur with sight.

Not long after we moved into this assisted living center, Peter became convinced I wasn't me; that I was a look-alike imposter. 'You can't fool me,' he said and he'd turn his head away and not look at me at all. (Tears roll down her face.) We've been married fifty years. Even when I know it is the disease, not him, it makes me feel so sad when he rejects me. - Jenny Ellis

Action: Jenny can try talking to him before she enters the room while she is still out of his sight. Because Capgras is only visual, Mr. Ellis should recognize this as his wife's voice. Then when she enters the room, his brain will automatically connect the voice he knows with the person and be more likely to "see" her as his wife and not an impostor.

Poor Hand-Eye Coordination

LBD patients tend to have more difficulty coordinating their vision with their hand movements than do other dementia patients. Therefore, many neurologists use a clock test to help with diagnosis. The patient draws a clock and points are given for correctness. The lower the points, the higher the probability of LBD.

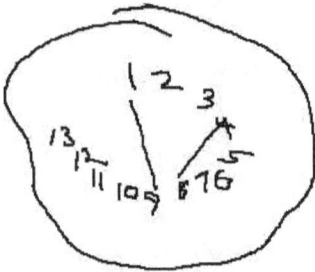

Simulated results of Mr. Dupree's clock test.

The clock test was one that Jake's physician used to help him decide that they were dealing with DLB rather than Alzheimer's. He lost points for the irregular circle, for having the numbers bunched in the middle, for the 13th number and for the placement of the hands. His score indicated an increased probability of LBD.

Poor Depth Perception

A patient with poor depth perception will perceive a change in texture as a change in height. He will also misjudge distances between themselves and others. The support group discussed their loved one's depth perception issues.

I notice that every once in a while David lifts his feet as though he's climbing stairs when he goes from the vinyl floor of our kitchen to our carpeted living room - Marie Newman

Mom always does. Of course, she's had PDD for several years. She was bumping into the furniture, door frames and even other people before she got her wheelchair. Well, she still does but not as much with the wheelchair. - Marion

Peter fell when he was reaching for a table and misjudged the distance. That's what put him in the hospital and started his downward slide. - Jenny Ellis

I've started filling Jake's coffee cup only about half full. He doesn't shake, it's just that he misjudges where the cup is and tips it over when he reaches for it. - Norma Dupree

These are all visuospatial issues, that of matching what you see with the space it actually occupies.

18. Other Sense Related-Symptoms

hyposmia: loss of the sense of smell.

taste buds: sensory sites in the mouth that identify sweet, salty, sour, bitter and savory.

***

Although visual perceptions seem to be most common with LBD, there are a few other sense-related symptoms as well.

Hallucinations Other Than Visual

Although visual hallucinations are so frequent with DLB that they are one of the core symptoms, other hallucinations can occur too. Of these, auditory hallucinations are the most common, appearing for about a third of those with either kind of LBD.[31]

Jake sometimes wakes me up because he's sure he heard a telephone. I answer the phone but no one is ever there! And he hears people knocking on our door too. He won't settle down until I answer the door and show him no one is there. Sure messes up my sleep! - Norma Dupree

Others may have "presence" hallucinations, where the patient has a sense that someone or something is near but just out of sight, maybe right behind them. Taste and touch hallucinations are comparatively rare.

Smell hallucinations are also uncommon. However they can be informally predictive of PDD.

My sister hasn't been able to smell for years but lately she's been complaining of a "stinky" smell in the house and keeps bugging me to find what's causing it. - Ellen

An impaired sense of smell is an early indicator of PD. Miss Cleary's unwelcome "smell" is likely a hallucination—and an early indicator of eventual dementia. Caregivers of patients with PDD often report that their loved one's first sign of dementia was the apparent return of their sense of smell via hallucinations.

Loss Of The Sense Of Smell

Greater than 95% of those living with PD lose their sense of smell.[32] This loss often occurs decades prior to the appearance of motor symptoms and thus smell tests are suggested as one way to predict this disease. The 2017 DLB diagnostic criteria now includes hyposmia, or loss of smell, as a symptom of DLB as well. Again, it can be a very early symptom, occurring well before cognitive symptoms do.

Since the sense of smell is highly involved in one's ability to taste, this loss affects a person's enjoyment of food and often changes their choices. Taste buds actually only pick up "sweet, salty, sour, bitter or savory." The sense of smell combines with taste to make the flavors that cause sweet chocolate to smell different than a melon or a vanilla cookie.

The sweet taste is often the strongest. Thus it is the one that can still give some enjoyment when smell is gone. That is why sweets make such great distractions and bribes.

Action. Use sweets as distractions and bribes when trying to move a person living with LBD away from a disruptive belief or behavior.

19. Sleep Disorders

excessive daytime sleep (EDS): persistent sleepiness and often a general lack of energy, during the day after apparently adequate or even prolonged nighttime sleep.

muscle atonia: restrained muscle activity, except middle ear muscle activity and eye movement.

REM sleep: Rapid Eye Movement sleep. The phase of sleep when a person dreams and when only the eyes can move.

REM sleep behavior disorder (RBD): A Lewy body-related disorder that causes loss of muscle atonia during REM sleep.

Active Dreams: A care partner's descriptive name for RBD, widely used in this and other Whitworth books.

***

Sleep problems are common with most dementias but are even more prevalent with LBD. Lewy bodies interfere with a person's ability to maintain good sleep habits, just as they interfere with a person's ability to maintain good cognition.

The two most prominent issues appear to be at odds with each other:

- REM sleep behavior disorder (RBD), or Active Dreams as care partners like to call it, which disturbs sleep.
- Excessive daytime sleeping (EDS) or too much sleep.

However, both are easily within the realm of those behaviors common to LBD: One is a vivid but not real visual experience; the other involves mental slowness.

LBD slows down most physical as well as mental functions. Therefore, it is not surprising that insomnia, although common in Alzheimer's, is uncommon with this disease. On the other hand, restless leg syndrome (RLS) is often present with LBD but unrelated.

REM Sleep Behavior Disorder (RBD)

During dreams, a natural muscle atonia (muscle restraint) occurs that makes it impossible for the normal body to move even during the most violent sequences. Only the eyes move and they do so rapidly, thus the name: rapid eye movement (REM) sleep.[33] When Lewy bodies damage the chemical switch that turns the muscle restraint on, the dreamer is able to move freely. They can physically act out their dreams, talk, move limbs about or even express violence towards a bed partner.

Sleep-walking and sleep-talking, while common with RBD, can also occur during non-REM sleep, i.e., when the patient is asleep but isn't dreaming. These behaviors are common with children but not with LBD.

Active Dreams may begin many, many years before any signs of dementia, making it one of the earliest Lewy body related symptoms. Over half of those living with RBD will develop some form of Lewy body disease.

Peter has never been a violent man when awake but his Active Dreams frightened me well before he was diagnosed with PD. Once I woke up just before his fist slammed into the side of my head. I screamed and apparently interrupted his dream because he just rolled over and went into a more restful sleep. - Jenny Ellis

The Ellises never connected the dreams with his illness or reported them to his doctor and none of his physicians asked Jenny about them until after his post-surgery degeneration.

In the morning I confronted Peter about trying to beat me up but he had no recollection of the incident. - Jenny Ellis

As with Mr. Ellis, Active Dreamers seldom remember anything about their behavior upon awakening. Thus, identifying the presence of this symptom requires a witness.

I've often wondered if my sister ever had Active Dreams. She certainly reacted to pain medications with hallucinations and delusions. - Ellen

Miss Cleary, a long time PD patient, is a prime candidate for Active Dreams. However, with only her cat as a sleeping partner no one could tell if she had experienced them or not. Knowledge of its presence might have led Miss Cleary's physicians to opt against her cancer surgery or use different pain medications.

Treatment

Just as a patient's symptoms will not be like anyone else's, their most appropriate treatment may not be either. With RBD, the first step is to make sure the patient is safe. Next, there are many non-drug remedies to try before you consider drugs. Drugs can be helpful but can also be problematic. Used with the drugs, these non-drug remedies will still be helpful and will often decrease the amount of drug required for an effect.

Physical Safeguards

Active Dreams can be so active that patient may fall out of bed or sleep-walk. Therefore, treatment starts with making the sleeping environment safer.

Move unsafe objects away from the bedside. Move those that could cause injury out the way.

Pad heavy or harder to move objects, such as the headboard.

Move the bed away from windows and/or block them with immovable objects such as a heavy dresser.

Have carpeted floors or padding next to the bed.

Bed partner safety. Bed partners may need to move to a different bed or even a different room.

Non-Drug Management

Avoid alcohol, especially in the evening. It interferes with a person's sleep cycle.

David hated to give up his evening glass of wine but when he did, he had fewer dreams. I was about to move to a different bed and if they come back later, I may still have to although I hate to disrupt the family. With the kids still at home this isn't easy, you know. On the other hand, the kids are great help when David needs to be calmed down. - Marie Newman

Review the patient's medication list. Behavior management and other anticholinergic drugs may trigger Active Dreams.

Limit excitement. Violent stimuli such as crime shows on TV often trigger Active Dreams but so can an exciting ball game.

Increase physical exercise in the morning and early afternoon. Limit it near bedtime when it can have the same effect as too much excitement.

Be alert for physical and emotional stress. Anxiety causing situations or illness such as a urinary tract infection can instigate or increase Active Dreams.

The best thing we did was that I started getting enough sleep! Our health aide was right on. Jake wasn't so perceptive before but now he reflects my every emotion. If I'm upset so is he—and then he acts it out in his sleep. - Norma Dupree

As Norma discovered, you need to be aware of the care partner's possible stress as well as the patient's. Both can trigger the patient's LBD symptoms.

Medical Management

Dementia drugs are often all that is needed at first. These act to decrease most LBD-related symptoms but as brain cells die, they lose their effectiveness and another drug may be needed.

I guess we are lucky. Hilda has had DLB for over 3 years now and no Active Dreams. And no hallucinations since she started on Aricept. - Barney Darnell

The Aricept may or may not be preventing the Active Dreams. If it is, it and the hallucinations both will likely show up as her dementia increases and the dementia drugs stop being effective.

Melatonin is a dietary supplement often used to improve sleep. It has been found to reduce or eliminate Active Dreams in some cases with few side effects. This is often the initial treatment of choice for the LBD patient.

We use melatonin for Jake's Active Dreams. At first I was giving it wrong. I thought I'd wait until he got restless and then give it. Wow! It really played havoc with his sleep cycles--and it didn't really help his dreaming. Instead, he started sleeping more during the day. But when the doctor's nurse explained that I should be giving it early in the evening, it actually started working. Well, that and now I take a nap when he does during the day. - Norma Dupree

Melatonin acts to adjust a person's sleep/wake cycle. It must be given at least an hour prior to sleep to be effective and, as Norma learned the hard way, should never be given to treat middle-of-the-night wakefulness.

Klonapin. When melatonin isn't enough, the doctor may suggest a small dose of Klonapin (clonazepam). A member of the benzodiazepine drug family, this drug should be used in low, cautious doses because it may increase confusion and sleepiness in elderly people.[34]

Atypical antipsychotic, such as Seroquel or Nuplazid. Nuplazid is newer and approved for use with Parkinson's with psychosis but is used off-label regularly for PDD and even DLB as well. However, it is quite expensive and thus, the doctor may opt to try something like Seroquel first, even though it is not only off-label but carries a warning about use with the elderly. Other atypicals may work but care partners find that Seroquel is least likely to cause serious side effects. One side effect is likely to be drowsiness, so it should be given in the evening.

Peter's neurologist put him on Seroquel for his combativeness and it helped the dreaming too. We did have to change his times so that he got his biggest dose in the evening. Now he's not napping as much during the day and sleeping better at night. - Jenny Ellis

Excessive Daytime Sleeping (EDS)

A person's brain is actually quite busy during sleep. This is when it transfers information from short to long term memory. It is also when it does its cleanup work, flushing out damaged cells and other "trash." With LBD, everything is slower and everything takes longer--if it gets done at all.

Excessive daytime sleeping (EDS) is the brain's way of working overtime to complete its normal nighttime work. A common LBD symptom, it is also associated with Alzheimer's, Parkinson's and most other neurological disorders. A person may feel compelled to nap repeatedly during the day or fall asleep at inappropriate times such as during meals. Sleeping well at night does not necessarily prevent daytime exhaustion or drowsiness.

During times of special interest or while doing things they especially enjoy, a person may be able to remain awake and alert. This is NOT a sign that he actually can control his sleeping, any more than "showtime" is evidence that patients can control when they do and do not function better than their normal.

EDS can be confused with overmedication. In fact, Lewy-savvy doctors will likely want to rule out medical concerns first by decreasing or changing any prescribed drugs with a sedative effect.

When I told Mom's geriatric psychiatrist about her 15 hours of sleep every night, he reduced some of her medication. But that didn't work. She began sleeping so poorly again at night that she slept even more during the day! When I reported that to the doctor, she nodded and said, "Well, now we know that isn't cause. Let's try something else." - Marion Peterson

Later, Marion did an informal survey of her online support group and found that with daytime naps included, 15 hours of sleep per day was not abnormal for LBD loved ones.

I've long thought that illness in and of itself requires extra sleep and certainly the efforts our loved ones put out to walk without falling, eat without choking and try their hardest to be normal must demand extra rest too. - Marion Peterson

She has a point. Add to this the general slowing down effect of LBD and it is no surprise that LBD patients spend much of their time sleeping.

EDS may also be connected to Active Dreams and the loss of rest they can cause. These more intense dreams may spill over into normal deep sleep cycle, cutting into the time the brain needs for its information transferring and janitoring jobs. Thus, the patient may be catching up on those missed tasks during daytime sleeping. Remember everything just takes longer. Even a good night's sleep still may not be enough to keep a patient from needing much more sleep during the day. Their body just seems to need more down time.

Treatment

Non Drug Management

Regular bedtime routine. Keep a regular bedtime and do everything you can to promote regular nighttime sleep.

While getting what should be enough sleep may not prevent EDS, poor sleep habits will definitely increase it. Work to improve these habits but at the same time, remember that the patient's brain may just need more down time to carry out its important sleep-related duties.

Regular, active daytime routine. Include exercise and social involvement.

Besides being a good deterrent for EDS, a regular and active routine is also just good care for any patient who might otherwise isolate in their room and stagnate.

I'm glad the staff here gets Mom out of her room every day and makes sure she has a chance to visit with other residents. She especially likes Sundays when they hold church and we all sing. Mom never could sing but she brightens up and doesn't act at all sleepy when there's singing going on. (Grin) But then she usually sleeps through the rest of the service. - Marion Peterson

Activities that trigger interest. Be sure to include activities that the patient especially enjoys doing, like past hobbies, etc. Make an effort to find out what a patient enjoys. Then try to provide it, whether it is singing, as with Mrs. Peterson, playing cards, scrapbooking, a special hobby or visiting with other residents. The family will perceive you as an integral part of the care team and a happy active patient is usually not only more cooperative but more alert.

Avoid daytime drugs with a sedative action. Check daytime drugs for sedative action and consult with their physician about changing their administration times to evening.

David didn't have EDS until his doctor started him on Seroquel. At first he was taking it in the mornings and then feeling drowsy a good share of the day. We changed it to evenings and now he doesn't have to nap at all sometimes. - Marie Newman

Avoid evening drugs that encourage alertness. Review evening drugs for action that might decrease nighttime sleep and consult with their physician about changing administration times to morning.

The doctor changed Jake's med times too. At first everything was divided up evenly between mornings and evenings. Now, he takes his cognition meds in the morning when he wants to be alert and awake and his Seroquel in the evenings. - Norma Dupree

Be alert for other issues that might cause sedation.

What worked for Mom was that the neurologist decreased her PD meds. That decreased her confusion but Mom also started sleeping less during the day. Of course, she can't move quite as well as she did but she was willing to accept the tradeoff. - Marion Peterson

EDS is not normally an early LBD symptom. When it is, the doctor usually looks for another, often drug-related reason. It can also be due to the time that the drug is given.

Hilda started sleeping a lot right after her diagnosis. Her doctor said her LBD wasn't so far advanced for her to sleep so much. Deciding it was probably due to being depressed, he prescribed an antidepressant. Hilda slept even more! Then the doc had her take them at night and voila! Hilda is not sleeping as much during the day and she's happier. We are also attending regular exercise class. I can tell when we miss a day. Hilda is much more likely to nap longer and be less responsive. - Barney Darnell

The doctor's guess that Hilda's sleeping might be due to depression was not a bad guess. It is a common LBD symptom, both clinically (due to the disease) and situationally.

Medical Management

Provigil. This drug is the medication of choice for EDS. It has also long been used as a brain booster for college students cramming for tests. With that in mind, it seems possible that it would also improve mental clarity with dementia. This has not been shown to be true, at least not over any length of time.

When Peter's doctor put him on Provigil for his daytime sleeping, she said it might improve Peter's cognition too. I didn't see much difference but he does stay awake more now. - Jenny Ellis

A word of caution. While Provigil can promote wakefulness, it is important to remember that the brain of a person living with dementia needs a great deal of sleep to do its work and stay healthy. Using drugs to promote wakefulness may deprive a person's brain of the sleep time it needs.

Address Active Dreams. Anything that allows a person to rest better at night may decrease EDS. It won't necessarily end it however.

Peter takes melatonin for his Active Dreams. The few active dreams he has now are much less violent. Peter always slept a lot in the daytime after he had a bad spell with RBD but now, without his violent dreams, he doesn't have to sleep in the daytime to recover from them. - Jenny Ellis

Restless Leg Syndrome (RLS)

This irritating syndrome can present alone or with many neurological diseases including LBD. While common with LBD, it is not a diagnostic symptom. With RLS, strong urges to move in order to stop painful or odd sensations can occur while the patient is asleep or awake. Like RBD, this syndrome may begin years before any other symptoms connected with dementia occur. However, it and RBD are not the same and should not be confused.[35]

Treatment

There is no cure for RLS and many of the drugs normally used to relieve RLS are contraindicated with LBD.

Non-Drug Management

The best preventions for RLS are non-medical:

Regular exercise. This increases blood flow.

Compression. Wrap legs in ace bandages or wear compression stockings or tight pantyhose.

Reduce caffeine, alcohol and tobacco use, particularly in the evening.

Medical Management

The following might be tried if approved by a physician and monitored closely for side effects:

- *Iron supplements.* Use only as ordered. Too much iron can cause liver and heart damage.

- *Anticonvulsants such as Neurontin (gabapentin)*. Side effects include excessive sleepiness and gait problems.
- *Opiates.* These narcotic drugs may cause psychotic symptoms such as delusions with LBD. Their addictive properties may cause a doctor to hesitate to prescribe them for long-term use.
- *Dopamine agonists,* such as Mirapex.[36] These are often the drug of choice for someone living with PD. However, when Lewy bodies enter the cognitive areas of the brain, the anticholinergic action of these drugs can cause confusion and other Lewy body symptoms.

These drugs should not be used with LBD.

- *Avoid Benzodiazepines*. Although these are sometimes prescribed for RLS, their strong anticholinergic drugs contradict their use with LBD. Their addictive properties may also cause a doctor to avoid prescribing them for long-term use.
- *Avoid Quinine.* This is sometimes used for leg cramps but is of little help with RLS. It can also have serious adverse reactions including death.[37]

To stop an RLS episode: Move the affected limb(s) for a few minutes. RLS is usually relieved by movement. If that doesn't work, apply heat or cold. A bath or soaking the feet in water may help. In bed, situate the patient on their side with a pillow between the knees.

Mom sometimes complains about RLS. Usually it's when she's in bed. I've found the best thing to do for her is to massage her legs. If that doesn't work then we go ahead and get her up and let her move around—a walk to the bathroom and back usually does the job. When we put her back to bed, I make sure she has pillows between her legs and settled so that she's really comfortable and ready to go back to sleep. - Marion Peterson

Marion recognizes that these hands-on remedies are safer than the medications and often just as successful. She could also take some preventative steps if the RLS occurs very often such as having her mother wear support hose during the day.

Insomnia

Insomnia is not a common LBD related issue but can occur due to LBD related issues such as depression or anxiety. A person's sleep may be interrupted by bad dreams or urinary problems. Their circadian rhythms, or natural sleep and wake rhythms, might be disrupted by other sleep related issues such as RLS or excessive daytime sleeping. They may wander instead of going back to bed after getting up to go to the bathroom. Medications given in the evening for cognition can sometimes cause wakefulness.

Primary caregivers *are* susceptible to insomnia.

Jake's dreams wake me up more than they do him. And then I have an awful time getting back to sleep. And Jake's dreams were getting worse. I talked to our health aide and she suggested I escape for a nap while she was here if I'd had a bad night. (Laugh) I complain about Jake and she wants to fix me! But it worked! With me happier and easier to live with, Jake's RBD is a lot better. - Norma Dupree

Although their loved ones may manage to fall asleep after an interruption, the caregivers have had to be more alert to provide help and maintain safety. Once their loved one is resettled they often find sleep avoiding them. This leads to fatigue-related irritability which is likely to increase dementia-related behaviors which in turn increases the caregiver's frustration. This causes a vicious cycle unless the sleep problems of both patient and caregiver are addressed.

Apnea

Sleep apnea,[38] also called sleep-disordered breathing (SDB), is a condition where sleepers stop breathing hundreds of times during the night. Apnea can happen with or without dementia. However, two LBD-related symptoms make it more likely:

- *Poor throat muscle control:* Obstructive sleep apnea occurs when the throat muscles relax and block the person's breathing.
- *ANS dysfunction:* Central sleep apnea occurs when the LBD-weakened autonomic nervous system doesn't deliver adequate signals from the brain to the muscles that control breathing and the person "forgets" to breathe.

A person may experience either obstructive or central apnea or both. The latter is called complex sleep apnea syndrome.

When the person "forgets" to breathe for whatever reason, the lack of oxygen in the brain wakes up the person and they start breathing again but they don't really catch up. With each waking event, the brain gets a little more behind. It needs lots of oxygen to fuel the janitorial service that works during sleep to clear out dementia-causing debris. With the brain still clogged, dementia symptoms can increase. (Think about how foggy you feel after a sleepless night!) Thus, it is a vicious circle. Dementia may cause apnea and then apnea may make the dementia worse!

Treatment

The first step in treatment is to differentiate between sleep apnea and Active Dreams. When lack of oxygen wakes up a person, a common reaction is to jerk and move one's limbs as if trying to ward off a breath-stopping attack. This physical activity gives the appearance of Active Dreams. Even a Lewy-savvy doctor may try to treat the sleep apnea prior to trying to decrease the Active Dreams.

CPAP mask. A continuous positive airway pressure (CPAP) mask is the treatment of choice for sleep apnea. This is an appliance that fits over the mouth and nose. It is connected to a pump which forces air into the nasal passages at pressures high enough to overcome obstructions in the airway and stimulate normal breathing. There are a variety of masks but they all must fit on the face and over the nose and mouth to work. The more automated the system, the easier it will be to use.

It is best to get this condition diagnosed and begin treatment as early as possible.

- If CPAP use becomes a habit before dementia appears or while it is mild, this formed habit may carry into the more severe dementia stages.
- If apnea is not identified and/or treated until after dementia is well entrenched, the patient will be less able to understand the need for the mask. Even if they could, they would also be less likely to tolerate this strange and annoying device without fussing or taking it off during sleep.

Doctors sometimes prescribe sedatives to help a person get to sleep initially while wearing the mask, but that is seldom an option for anyone with dementia, especially not anyone with LBD. A milder anti-psychotic like Nuplazid or a mild anti-depressant like Welbutrin might help, but they are not always an option either. Some people tolerate these drugs and some don't. Besides, waking up and going back to sleep--with the mask on--is the real hurdle. It can't be fixed over and over with drugs.

In an online forum, a care partner told of how disorienting it was for her loved one to wake up with this strange contraption on his face. Another group member responded, "At this point, I just wouldn't bother. There are enough things in that man's life to cause him panic, distress and discomfort without adding a CPAP mask." The group member has a point. The effort to keep the mask on can also be a distressing and often sleep-depriving effort for the care partner. Is a benefit limited because the mask comes off over and over worth the high cost in peace and sleep? Even if the patient is in a care facility, the staff effort may not be worth the results.

This may be an example of when the care team (care staff, physician and care partner) must stop and re-evaluate their goals. There comes a time in the care of a dementia patient when care goals must change from improving function to choosing comfort. A CPAP mask is actually very good for improving function--it can greatly improve clarity if used properly. But if the dementia is so advanced that they can't use it properly, it is probably more of a burden than a help.

The changing of a goal from function to comfort is not easy because it signals the beginning of the end. However, this change doesn't have to happen all at once. With each treatment and each activity, the care team gets to make a separate decision. Some efforts at maintaining function can last much longer than others. Using or not using a CPAP may simply be the first decision of this sort that comes along.

20. Mood Disorders

anxiety: A persistent feeling of being restless, tense or nervous.

apathy: A lack of motivation, an inability to initiate or care about anything and minimal feelings.

chronic depression: Depression brought on by a disease such as LBD.

depression: A persistent feeling of sadness and loss of interest in activities once enjoyed.

empathy deficit: An inability to put yourself in another's place and feel their emotions as your own yet know they are really that other person's.

situational depression: Depression brought on by life experiences such as a LBD diagnosis.

***

Empathy deficit, apathy, depression and anxiety are all LBD symptoms that can show up together or individually. They can be difficult to tell apart but that isn't usually important because they are treated much the same. As with all behavioral symptoms, the patient has no control over any of these symptoms.

Empathy Deficit

Empathy is an abstract thinking skill that requires a person to be able to see themselves and their feelings as separate from others.[39] LBD patients are experts at picking up feelings but instead if identifying them as the other person's they own them.

I was really angry about something that had happened at lunch. When I went into Mrs. Peterson's room, she picked up on that and started yelling at me. --Anna, health tech

Mrs. Peterson had no trouble picking up Anna's feelings but then she owned them and vented the anger at the nearest target, Anna.

Treatment

Monitor your feelings before entering the room of anyone living with dementia and present as positive an attitude as you can for the best cooperation. Drugs that treat cognitive symptoms may also improve a person's ability to empathize temporarily.

Apathy

You may recognize dopamine as a chemical in the brain that facilitates mobility. It also facilitates pleasure. When there is a lack of dopamine, apathy occurs, resulting muted feelings, a lack of motivation and an inability to initiate or care about anything.[40]

I fell and David didn't even notice. He just asked me to get him more coffee. He used to be so considerate and now he's just indifferent to anything but his own needs. In fact, he doesn't care about much of anything anymore. He used to love gardening and so I got out a seed catalog and started turning the pages and talking about the different plants and vegetables. He paid attention and even make a comment or two. -- Marie

David's apathy prevented him from showing any compassion. It also keeps him from initiating activities, but if Marie does, he can follow along and even find some enjoyment in them.

Treatment

Encourage care partners to remember that apathy's indifference "is the disease talking, not my loved one." If you initiate an activity, the patient may be able to mirror it. Make sure the activity isn't so demanding that it overwhelms instead helps. Music therapy and massage are safe non-drug interventions that may help.

PD drugs may decrease apathy but monitor for cognitive symptoms. Some antidepressants may be helpful, but they can also make the apathy worse and so monitor carefully.

Depression

Depression includes a feeling of ongoing sadness that interferes with life in general. It is usually accompanied by feelings of inadequacy, helplessness and and makes everything less enjoyable, more tiring and more difficult.[41] It can be chronic, caused by the lack of pleasure hormones like dopamine and serotonin. This type is understandably more common with LBD than with other dementias.

Performing tasks, making decisions or interacting with others all become more difficult. Since these are also skills affected by dementia, depression makes them even worse.

Hilda is still willing to go out for ice cream and such but she gets awfully sad. I've noticed that her periods of sadness often follow periods of clarity. -- Barney

Hilda's depression is likely situational, brought about by her temporary awareness of her illness. This type is common with all dementias and extremely common with care partners.

This disease is so overwhelming that I get depressed. There's times when it's all I can do to do what has to be done...and sometimes not even that! -- Marie

Marie is experiencing caregiver depression. If she doesn't get help soon, David will likely mirror her mood and the situation will only get worse.

Treatment

Non drug treatment for the care partner starts with finding a safe place such as a support group where she can vent and learn coping methods.

Non-drug interventions for depression of any kind include exercise, social interactions, adequate sleep and a pleasing environment. These should always be tried first and continued even if drugs are deemed necessary. Care partners and staff should also monitor their own moods and be sure to present as positive attitude as possible for the patient to mirror.

Mild antidepressants that are usually safe with LBD include drugs such as Zoloft (sertraline) and Lexapro (escitalopram).

Anxiety

Anxiety symptoms include feeling nervous, restless or tense and is more common with LBD than it is with other dementias, due to Lewy body-related changes in brain chemistry. However, it can also be related to a person's inability to deal with challenges due to cognitive

107

losses. It makes activities of daily living more difficult, reduces quality of life and leads to more frequent nursing home admission than for people living with dementia who don't experience anxiety.[42]

Mom has spells when she gets awfully restless. Since she's in a wheelchair, she can't move around a lot but she sure squirms. Sometimes, I can blame frustration but at other times, it just is. -- Marion, daughter of Laura Peterson

Mrs. Peterson appears to be exhibiting both types of anxiety, the more situational type and that caused by LBD.

Treatment

Non-drug treatments include removing frustrations and other irritants that can lead to anxiety, including too high expectations or tasks that are too difficult.

The newer antidepressants like those used for depression can also be helpful for anxiety. Anti-anxiety drugs or Haldol are not recommended for treating anxiety in anyone living with LBD. A doctor might prescribe a milder antipsychotic such as Seroquel (quetiapine) or Nuplazid (pimavanserin) in small doses for short periods of time.

21. Autonomic Nervous System Dysfunctions

autonomic functions: automatic functions, those that the brain controls without a person's conscious attention.

dehydration: A harmful reduction in the amount of water in the body.

dysphagia: Difficulty swallowing

fecal impaction: A large, hard mass of stool stuck in the colon or rectum that can't be pushed out.

orthostatic hypotension (OH): Low blood pressure upon rising.

✱✱✱

The Autonomic Nervous System affects all of the following organs and functions:

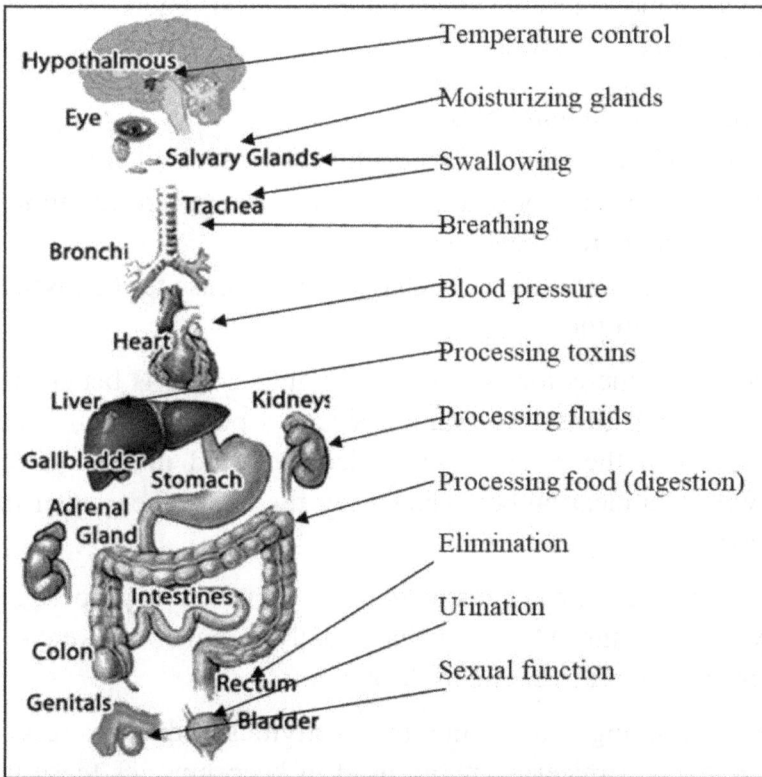

When Lewy bodies attack and weaken weaken the autonomic nervous system (ANS), its ineffectiveness causes the organs that it controls to be slower and less efficient, resulting in a variety of LBD-related symptoms. In retrospect some, such as constipation, may be the first LBD symptoms to appear.

General Treatment

Since these varied symptoms all stem from ANS dysfunction, some treatments are general and can prevent or address several different symptoms at once.

Non-Drug Management

Avoid dehydration. Getting enough fluids into a dementia patient can sometimes be difficult, due to issues like swallowing and the fear of incontinence. However, adequate fluid intake is highly important for preventing and treating all ANS symptoms and especially necessary for those involving the gastrointestinal and urinary (GI) tracts.

Dehydration:

- compromises the immune system.
- makes all GI and urinary tract dysfunctions more likely.
- decreases skin quality and makes urine stronger, resulting in skin irritations and pressure sores.
- can cause dementia-related behavior in response to the discomfort of any or all of the above.

  Action: Use urine color as a hydration guide. This is better than trying to count glasses of water because a person's fluid needs will vary with the person. With adequate fluid in the system, urine will be a clear amber. The darker the color, the greater the dehydration.

Exercise. Exercise helps the whole body to function properly. This definitely includes the ANS. Develop a daily regimen of exercise that challenges but doesn't overwhelm the patient.

Take time. Building extra time into activities reduces stress. The resulting relaxation releases energy used to keep muscles tense which the ANS can now use to improve functions such as swallowing and digestion. Because the patient tends to mirror their caregiver's mood, it is important that you work in a relaxed manner as well.

Make activities enjoyable. Besides improving quality of life, enjoyment promotes relaxation, which allows the various organs to function at their best. It also causes the release of "feel good" hormones that increase body functionality.

Adjust the bed. When the head of the bed is about four inches higher than the foot, it will help with several of the ANS dysfunctions, from orthostatic hypotension to constipation.

Medical Management

Dementia drugs. These are often all that is necessary at first. In fact, because so many of the medications regularly used with ANS dysfunctions may increase other LBD symptoms, these may be the only drugs that can be used.

Monitor for side effects. Many drugs can have a negative effect with the ANS in general or with a specific organ that it controls. Know the drugs a patient is taking and what their side effects are. Continually monitor for and report any that you notice. Although side effects can appear at any time as the patient's system changes, they are most likely at the start of a new medication. As the hands-on care provider, you may be the first person to notice any conflicts.

Specific Symptoms

The ANS controls a multitude of organs that function to keep a person healthy. The functions discussed here are the ones most commonly affected by Lewy bodies. When no drug treatment is mentioned, dementia drugs are usually the only ones used.

Temperature Regulation

Like a menopausal woman, LBD patients may feel hot then cold for no discernible reason. However, being cold is more common. Caregivers often report that their patient is always cold, sometimes even when the temperatures are in the 80's or above.

Treatment

Use layers. Help the patient to dress in easy-to-use layers. A lap rug or simple shrug that they can put on when cold and discard when warmer will increase comfort.

Avoid drafts. The LBD patient's internal heating system can't adjust well to deal with these.

Dysphagia

Dysphagia, or difficulty in swallowing, [43] is very common. Fluids are the most difficult to swallow but eating in general may also become a challenging task. Insufficient fluids leads to dehydration. This causes a variety of ANS system dysfunctions, such as urinary retention, to be even worse. Poor eating habits or not eating enough may lead to malnutrition, which decreases immunity and health in general.

Choking is an immediate reaction to dysphagia and can be quite serious. Aspiration of liquids into the lungs can result in an infection which can turn into pneumonia. Pneumonia is a major cause of death with LBD patients. In addition, choking uses up energy and decreases quality of life.

When Mom has difficulty swallowing, she gets a lot of saliva in her mouth and drools, which embarrasses her. It makes me worry about her choking. - Marion Peterson

Marion's concerns are valid. Saliva secretion is a normal part of the swallowing process, providing the lubrication for food to slip more easily down the esophagus. When the swallowing process is weak, the saliva backs up and that's when Mrs. Peterson drools. Even worse, she may also choke on the backed up saliva.

Some of Mom's medications cause dry mouth. I'm always giving her ice chips. This helps her speech and it's good for her constipation too. - Marion Peterson

This is just the opposite of the saliva problem but it can also make swallowing difficult. Mrs. Peterson does need some fluid. For her the ice chips work because they melt slowly enough that only a small amount must be swallowed at a time.

It is becoming difficult for Peter to swallow water and he can't deal with ice chips at all; he does better with juices and other thicker liquids. - Jenny Ellis

Mr. Ellis' response to ice chips is more common than Mrs. Peterson's. Their extreme cold is more likely than not to trigger choking. As with everything involved with LBD, this is trial and error.

Thick liquids are easier to swallow than water. However, this is another area of trial and error. Some people prefer only lightly thickened fluids. Others may require "pudding-thick" liquids, which are usually eaten with a spoon. Even these thicker liquids work to provide one's daily quota of fluid.

Treatment

Use a dysphagia cup. This specially-designed cup makes it easier to swallow when one's neck is not extended. The high back rim of this cup allows a person to sip and swallow without throwing one's head back. The large handle makes it easier for a patient to hold.

Positioning. Keep the patient in a sitting or upright position during the meal and for 15 to 30 minutes afterwards to facilitate the passage of the food from the throat into the stomach.

Make dinner time fun. Besides the fact that the relaxation from enjoyment makes the ANS function better, it also improves motivation. Eating can be hard and sometimes, scary work. If the patient likes the person feeding him and enjoys his meal, he will be more willing to make the effort to eat.

Use brightly colored plates that contrast with the food colors. These are easier for a person with poor visual perceptions to see.

Avoid distractions. A dementia patient has difficulty multitasking so his attention will be on the distraction, not the eating.

Avoid extreme food temperatures. Foods that are too hot or too cold may be unpleasant to a dementia patient, triggering gagging and choking.

Use reminders. You may need to remind the patient to chew or swallow. Otherwise, the food may ball up in the patient's cheeks and lead to choking when swallowing is finally attempted.

Use thickened liquids as needed. As the dysphagia increases, you will need to thicken "thin" fluids like water, tea, coffee, milk and broth. Use natural thickeners such as cornstarch or potato flakes or you can buy commercial thickeners from a variety of sources.

Be alert for choking. Be especially alert with anything that melts or turns to liquid in the mouth such as ice cream, ice cubes or juicy fruits like oranges or watermelon.

Avoid straws. The position of the head required and the sucking action itself can lead to choking.

Orthostatic Hypotension (OH)

Blood gets to the brain via the bloodstream. When a person's blood pressure is too low, the heart can't pump an adequate supply of oxygen-carrying blood up to the brain. Without adequate oxygen in the brain, a person will become dizzy and can even pass out.

When a person rises from a horizontal position, blood naturally begins to pool in the lower extremities, decreasing the amount of blood available for the heart to pump. This results in lower blood pressure without the power necessary to pump needed oxygenated blood to the brain. Normally, the ANS immediately constricts the blood vessels and this allows the pressure to return to normal.

With a dysfunctional ANS, this adjustment still occurs but it is too slow, resulting in inadequate oxygen in the brain. OH, or low blood pressure upon rising, occurs in as many as 20% of persons with PD and increases to 50-60% of persons with LBD.[44]

When a person with OH rises from a bed or chair, symptoms such as dizziness or fainting occur. In most cases the greatest danger lies in the falls and injuries that occur when a dizzy, unstable patient attempts to move around unaided.

Occasionally syncope, with coma-like symptoms can occur. OH can be lethal. If the slowness is extreme, the body may be unable to adjust in time to keep the heart beating and death can occur.

You may have experienced a mild form of these symptoms after a surgery, which often interferes with ANS function. When you sat up, you probably felt dizzy and had to "dangle" or sit on the side of the bed for a few minutes before the nurse would let you get up. The difference between this and LBD is that surgery-related OH is temporary. As the body recovers after surgery, so does ANS function.

Treatment

There are some drugs that treat OH but due to the danger of drug-drug or LBD-drug interactions, non-drug options should be tried first.

Non-Drug Management

Wait period. Raise up slowly to allow the ANS time to work. For the surgery patient, a few minutes might be enough between rising and walking but for the person living with LBD, the time could be 10 minutes or more.

If Jake takes his time getting up, he's good for the rest of the morning. If he doesn't, he gets dizzy and I know he'd fall if he tried to walk. In fact, he almost did a few days ago. I helped him sit up and told him to sit there while I got his robe. As soon as my back was turned he tried to walk. I hate to think what would have happened if I hadn't been close enough to catch him before he fell! - Norma Dupree

Supervision. With the inability to understand reasons for safety or control impulses, a person living with LBD requires supervision to keep them from moving too quickly.

While Jake is sitting on the side of the bed I have him do some exercises. This gives him something to do and makes the time go faster. - Norma Dupree

Physical exercises. These will cause one's muscles to assist the ANS to work properly. Start with straight leg raises while lying down or knee extensions while seated. Then, while sitting, wiggle/raise toes and cross/uncross legs.

Sodium. Adequate salt in the diet maintains blood pressure, which may decrease OH. The physician may even prescribe salt tablets to assure that the patient is getting enough sodium. However, extra salt can raise normal blood pressure and should not be given without a physician's advice.

115

Avoid prolonged bed rest. When the body lies prone, the blood spreads evenly throughout the body. The longer the time spent in bed, the more this happens and the more difficult it is for a damaged ANS to adjust.

Head elevation. Sleep with the head elevated. It helps the body to maintain more blood in the upper regions and decreases the amount of "orthostatic stress," or the body's need to adjust to normal blood pressure.

Use compression stockings. This keeps more blood in the upper body, closer to the heart. This is one of the most difficult options to continue, because the constriction may not be comfortable, especially until one becomes used to it. Without the ability to understand cause and effect, being uncomfortable has no value and isn't tolerated well!

Medical Management

Medication review. The physician's first action is usually to review existing prescriptions and adjusting any that have side-effects that might be causing OH. For the person living with PDD, this may be an anti-parkinsonian drug, such as Eldepryl (selegiline).

ProAmatine (midodrine). This drug raises blood pressure by constricting blood vessels and does so continually, without respect to need, while it is in the bloodstream. Because OH is not continual, this drug can result in drug-related high blood pressure but its short action makes this less of a problem. It should not be given within 4 hours of bedtime so that it won't conflict with bedtime drugs. A good time to give it is when the patient is sitting on the side of their bed waiting to get up.

Mestinon (pyridostigmine). This drug has an action that responds to the body's orthostatic stress and works only when the blood pressure is too low. While Mestinon tends to works best for OH, it is fairly mild and is sometimes combined with ProAmatine for increased effectiveness.

Constipation And Fecal Incontinence

A defective ANS tends to slow the digestive process, which can result in constipation, a symptom usually associated with all LB diseases. However, episodes of diarrhea can be a side effect of the cognition medication or may follow efforts to solve the constipation problem. As the disease progresses, fecal incontinence becomes more likely especially at times when the stool is not solid and is therefore harder for the rectal sphincter to hold back.

Severe constipation[45] can cause severe bloating, abdominal pain, nausea/vomiting and headaches. In addition, there may be what appears to be mild diarrhea. This is actually a small amount of stool that has been able to seep out from around the blockage.

Treatment

Prevention

A high-fiber diet. This holds fluid in the bowel and increases gastric motility. Consider commercial compounds such as Metamucil or Fruit-eze if you have trouble getting the patient to eat enough natural fiber.

Small frequent meals rather than two or three large meals a day. The patient's damaged digestion system processes at a slower rate than a normal system. It processes frequent small amounts of food more easily than large, less frequent amounts.

Prune juice. This works well as a natural gentle laxative for many patients.

Adequate fluids and exercise to keep the body working well.

Regular bathroom routine. Be especially alert when this routine is broken, as with travel.

Daily preventative routine of stool softeners/osmotic laxatives. (See Treatment, below, for description) May only need these every other day or so. (This varies with the individual. Too much can lead to diarrhea.)

Medical Management

All treatment should be discussed with the patient's physician. Although a treatment may be safe in most cases, LBD patients are sensitive-prone and are often on other, possibly conflicting, drugs. Even when the treatment appears safe and helpful, it should be monitored carefully since the disease is always progressing and the patient's response may change.

Avoid dopamine antagonists such as Reglan, which are sometimes used to decrease PD drug caused nausea and vomiting. These are NOT considered safe to use with LBD and may have similar side effects as Haldol.

Stool softeners. These hold fluid in the bowel and soften stools. They are gentle and can be used regularly with little problem.

Osmotic laxatives, such as Miralax. These are stool softeners with an added mild laxative effect. These are gentle enough that they can be used even with LBD but as with all drugs, should be used only with a doctor's approval.

Avoid most other laxatives. These stronger drugs are more likely to cause loss of body fluids and potassium due to diarrhea. They are not usually recommended and should only be used when advised to do so by the physician.

Enema. If constipation becomes severe, enemas may be necessary. These should not be used unless all other efforts have been tried. However, poor muscle control and poor understanding of the need for this often uncomfortable procedure can make this unsuccessful with LBD.

Suppositories. These are usually not very helpful for the same reasons that enemas are not.

Impaction removal: If the constipation gets very bad, you may need to try to excavate it by hand. Since the rectal area is tender, this requires knowledge of how to do the process safely. Care staff are usually trained to handle severe constipation and impactions but care partners may not be.

Hospital emergency room. When a patient lives at home, an ER visit is likely the first option once an impaction is suspected unless a care partner knows what they are doing. Severe constipation is painful and possibly deadly if not dealt with quickly.

Diarrhea And Fecal Incontinence

With the use of cognition medications, constipation may turn to diarrhea.

It can be difficult for the person with full cognitive and physical abilities to deal with diarrhea. With limited cognitive abilities and limited sphincter control, fecal incontinence may become as common as urinary incontinence and can be more difficult to deal with.

Mom is often constipated. I can tell when she needs a laxative because she gets more confused. But then, it gets worse. Even the gentle laxatives make it hard for Mom to get to the bathroom in time. And then she tries to do her own cleaning up. What a mess! Once, not long before she went into Anytown, I had to clean up the whole wall where Mom had wiped her hands. (Sigh) And then I put Mom into the shower, clothes and all. - Marion

At times like this, it can be easy for the caregiver to forget that the dementia patient is not deliberately trying to be difficult. Marion's mom was doing the best she could. Her accidents and the way she deals with them are not in her control.

Treatment

Non-Drug Management

Routine. Developing a patient-specific toileting regimen to fit those times when a bowel movement was most likely in the past may help to eliminate fecal incontinence.

Adult diapers, such as Depends. These may help to contain the problem. However, clean the patient as quickly as possible to avoid infections from fecal contamination.

Fiber compounds, such as Metamucil. These work to keep the elimination regular, which addresses diarrhea as well as constipation.

Good hygiene. This helps to avoid the spread of infectious diarrhea.

Medical Management

Dosage adjustment. Check with the physician to see if the patient's cognition drugs need to be decreased or changed.

Imodium. This is the over-the counter drug of choice for diarrhea. A mild anticholinergic, it should be used sparingly. Start with no more than a half-dose and monitor carefully.

Non-anticholinergic drugs, such as Flomax. These are sometimes also prescribed for fecal incontinence.

Sexual Dysfunction

Erectile dysfunction may be due to ANS dysfunction or to dementia in general. This can result in low self-esteem in the early LBD patient. Impotence or other sexual dysfunctions can reduce personal contact, such as hugging and general touching.

Other roadblocks to marital intimacy include the patient's paranoia, accusations and aggressive demands. These may replace prior qualities of warmth, caring, humor or playfulness. Forgetfulness may lead to excessive demands for sex and poor hygiene may make the act unattractive to the partner. Eventually, the dementia patient will lose any interest in sex.[46]

An LBD patient's lack of impulse control and judgment can also lead to sexual inappropriateness.

Mr. Ellis gets all amorous sometimes. He tries to pat my backside if I stand too close and he even spoke up once and invited me into bed with him. I've found that ignoring him—and keeping out of his way is the best solution. - Anna, care technician

Treatment

Non-Drug Management

Ignore inappropriate behavior, then redirect. This is not something the patient can control.

Sexual enjoyment that does not include intercourse can be substituted. Hugging, kissing and touching remain important even when intercourse is not.

Medical Management

Especially with the younger patient, where this may be an issue, erectile dysfunction can be treated with drugs such as sildenafil, tadalafil or vardenafil taken by mouth. However, most caregivers report little need for medical intervention.

22. Urinary Tract Dysfunctions

urinary tract: the body organs that produce, store and discharge urine, including kidneys, ureters, bladder and urethra.

UTI: Urinary tract infection

urinary retention: The inability to completely empty one's bladder. May also be the inability to start urination or once started, the inability to fully empty the bladder.

urinary incontinence: Lack of voluntary control of urination. Inability to control the urinary sphincter.

***

Urinary tract dysfunctions are at least partly a result of ANS dysfunctions. However, there are also other issues involved.

General Treatment

Prevention

The general treatment suggestions for ANS dysfunctions are equally important with urinary tract dysfunctions:

- adequate hydration
- adequate exercise
- a relaxed, patient manner
- continual monitoring

Good personal hygiene. It is important to keep the whole diaper area clean for several reasons:

- Fecal matter can block the urinary tract, resulting in urinary retention.
- E. coli, a common bacteria found in fecal matter, can enter the urinary tract and cause infections.
- Strong acidic urine left on the skin can cause irritations and sores.

Medical Management

Dementia drugs may improve ANS function enough to solve urinary problems such as poor sphincter control.

Urinary Retention

This occurs in over a third of those with LBD.[47] Urinary retention occurs when the ANS slows the passage of fluids through the body and the urine backs up like a stagnant pond without a proper outlet. These backed up fluids become an incubator for bladder infections, which can lead to kidney damage and even death.

Mom resists drinking her water. She finds the bathroom trips just too tiring and this is her way of avoiding them. - Marion Peterson

Drinking less water actually triggers the need to urinate even more. The lower pressure from less fluid makes the kidneys work even harder-- with less result. Of course, Mrs. Peterson is beyond understanding this. She isn't able to get past her "what doesn't go in won't need to come out" principle.

Mrs. Peterson's inadequate fluid intake causes other problems too. Adequate hydration is especially important for a variety of reasons, including better ANS management of sphincters and kidneys.

Treatment

Non-Drug Management

Stimulate voiding:

- Sit the patient in a warm bath, or under a warm shower if bathing is not possible.
- Run water in a sink, shower or bathtub within sight and hearing of the patient.

Medical Management

Urecholine or Duvoid (bethanechol) This is the usual drug of choice for urinary retention and is recommended for use with LBD.[48] However, like all drugs, it should be used cautiously and monitored carefully.

Catheterization. This may be needed if retention becomes painful. Catheterization should be done by someone trained to do it so as to prevent damage to the urinary tract.

Incontinence

Although incontinence is almost universal in all dementias, ANS dysfunction decreases one's ability to control the urinary sphincter. A patient can develop infections or pressure sores if not kept clean. Incontinence can also result in embarrassment for the early and mid-stage LBD patient and can increase isolation by limiting their willingness to leave the home.

Mom quit going to church when she became incontinent. I tried to get her to use Depends and go anyway but she was too embarrassed. I'm glad they have church services here at Bridgestone. Mom feels comfortable attending here with others who have her same issues. - Marion Peterson

Incontinence also increases the chances of skin infections, especially if there is accompanying dehydration to make the urine stronger than usual.

Peter's been incontinent since he came out of the hospital with his broken hip. I'm so thankful that the aides here keep him cleaned up and work to avoid skin infections." Jenny Ellis

Treatment

Non-Drug Management

Schedule toileting. Scheduled voiding regimens may help even with the patient whose dementia is more advanced. Require the patient to go to the bathroom every two hours whether they feel a need or not.

Use cues. Reinforce environmental cues by doing things like putting signs or labels on the toilet.

Simplify clothing so that it is easy to undress for toileting.

Use adult diapers. This may eliminate some of the embarrassment a patient may initially feel about incontinence.

Monitor carefully. Check for physical problems like an infection or hidden injury. Some patients become incontinent when anything else is wrong just as some develop behavior problems.

To avoid bedtime incontinence:

Limit evening drinking. While adequate water is still important, stopping water intake two hours before bedtime may help bedtime incontinence.

Raised legs in the evening and/or support hose. These both keep fluids from pooling in the lower extremities and traveling back to the bladder after the patient lies down for the night.

Treat sleep apnea. Sleep apnea[49] is common with most dementias. It can inhibit the production of a hormone secreted during sleep that acts as an anti-diuretic. It also tends to trigger the kidneys to excrete fluids.

Medical Management

Avoid bladder control drugs such as Dridase or Ditropan (oxybutynin), Detrol LA (tolterodine) or Vesicare (solifenacin). These commonly used bladder control drugs are anticholinergics. These drugs compete with the medications used for cognition. (Some caregivers have reported success with Vesicare but it should be used only with a physician's direction and careful monitoring.)

Non-anticholinergic drugs. Drugs like Flomax (tamsulosin) and Proscar (finasteride) usually have fewer side effects with LBD.

Avoid Hytrin (terazosin). Although this not an anticholinergic, it lowers blood pressure. This makes it a poor choice for someone with LBD.

Urinary Tract Infection (UTI)

This is often a secondary symptom resulting from urinary retention, poor personal hygiene or both which can be made worse by incontinence. However, as LBD progresses, UTIs become such a fact of life that it becomes difficult to identify a specific cause. Left untreated, UTIs can become major health problems.

Symptoms include pain and burning upon urination, a need to urinate repeatedly without much success, nausea/vomiting and blood in the urine. Sometimes there are no symptoms at all. Sometimes there may be symptoms but the patient is unable to recognize them as such or communicate about them even if they do. The most common symptom for some dementia patients is dementia-related behaviors, often hallucinations or agitation.

Our health aide and I are continually trying to get more fluids down Jake. Sometimes he just gets too tired and pushes the cup away and won't drink anymore. Last week Jake was awfully weak. I knew he was getting dehydrated so I called paramedics. As soon as Jake saw the white coats on the paramedics he began cussing me and trying to hit me. They took him to the ER where he got IV fluids and did tests that showed that he had a UTI. - Jenny Ellis

Jenny's concern was valid. Not only her husband's weakness but his unusually violent behavior were signals that something was likely wrong.

I wasn't surprised about the UTI—that's why he was acting-out so badly. Of course, the people at the ER wanted to give him Haldol. This time, I had my LBDA Wallet Card ready and they gave him something else instead. And they started treatment for the UTI. Jake's home now and acting a lot better. - Norma Dupree

The above scenario is played out often with LBD patients and their care partners. Retention and dehydration combine to cause a UTI; the patient acts out in reaction to the discomfort and ends up in the emergency room where the staff may or may not know how to treat someone with LBD.

Haldol is an inexpensive but efficient drug for controlling agitated patients and is used as such in many hospital emergency rooms. However, it is also a very strong anticholinergic and likely to trigger severe sensitivity reactions with LBD. This knowledge isn't as common in emergency rooms as the Haldol is! Norma's wallet card saved the day. Encourage every care partner to obtain and carry one if they will be taking their loved one to any medical facility besides those known to be familiar with that patient and with LBD.

Treatment

Prevention

General treatment suggestions for ANS dysfunctions. See first of chapter.

Prevent/treat urinary retention, which if left untreated, can lead to URIs.

Cranberry juice. This acidic juice[50] has an active ingredient that can stop bacteria, particularly E. coli, from sticking to the bladder wall. This can help to lessen the occurrences of UTIs. However, the ingredient is not strong enough to be of use as a cure-all. Cranberry juice must be considered as part of the caregiver's UTI fighting arsenal, not the whole answer.

Medical Management

An LBD patient's urinary tract infections can be treated the same as those of any elderly person.

Antibiotics are usually prescribed with the direction that all of the prescription must be consumed. Using the medication only until the patient feels better may result in a resistance to that drug that will make it ineffective the next time it is used.

The Behaviors

Managing dementia-related behaviors is one of the most difficult parts of dementia care. You need to know these basic facts before you can successfully manage the behavior of a dementia patient:

Security is critical: For the dementia patient, maintaining control of their ever-changing lives is essential. Change, any loss of the known or the absence of a trusted care partner feels life-threatening.

Emotions rule. When thinking abilities fade, emotions, usually the stronger, more insistent negative ones, take over. (Review the chapters on emotions (Chapter 2) and thinking errors (Chapter 11).

Comfort is key: Anything that adds positive feelings, especially comfort and security, will decrease the negative emotions that lead to behaviors.

Here and now is all there is. Only that which can be personally experienced in the moment counts. The past and future are concepts no longer understood.

Once you understand the basics, you can begin trying to manage the behaviors:

Ignore non-disruptive behaviors. If a behavior bothers the care person but not the patient, only the care person needs to change.

Reduce triggers: Triggers can be environmental, physical or emotional but are always forms of discomfort.

Empathy, acceptance and apologies are magic. These help the patient to feel heard, which make responses to dementia-related behaviors more successful.

Behavior management drugs offer mixed blessings. They can be helpful but should be used sparingly and with careful monitoring.

Note from the authors:

When we updated this book, we discovered how much we'd learned about behavior management since it was first written. While the information in this section will help you deal with these baffling, frustrating and confusing behaviors, it is only a start.

Responsive Dementia Care: Fewer Behaviors Fewer Drugs provides you with over 300 pages of evidence-based and care- partner-tested information, examples and suggestions for understanding and managing dementia-related behaviors. It is available on our website, LBDtools.com and Amazon.

23. Basics

dementia-related behaviors: Those behaviors brought on by dementia or by a dementia-related symptom.

security: Feeling safe and in control

familiarity: Provides security because a patient knows what to expect.

response: A thought out action.

reaction: Acting without thought.

comfort: A positive feeling that results when there is little stress.

change: A removal of the familiar and a threat to security.

routine: Doing something the same way every time.

here and now: the present, with no reference to past or present.

going home: feeling like I did when I didn't have dementia.

***

Security Is Critical

Dementia continually causes losses for anyone living with dementia: loss of skills, loss of understanding, loss of awareness, loss of so many things. For the person living with LBD, there are physical losses as well. Therefore, the patient tends to cling to those things they still recognize, the people they still know, the things they can still do and the routines that make it easier to know what to do next.

Familiarity, not variety. Where once variety and a challenge of one's skills was fun and entertaining, it is now experienced as a loss of control and thus, feels threatening and scary.

Sameness is the name of the game. The same food, the same clothes, the same routine day after day feels safe. Stick with the familiar. Buy the same color and style of clothes. Go to the same places. Do the same things. Variety isn't fun anymore.

Status quo, not change. Change threatens to remove the familiarity of the old, comfortable things and activities along with their accompanying feelings of security. Once a welcome challenge, change is now overwhelming and uncomfortable. Now the challenge is simply to maintain the status-quo.

Jake used to love to try new things, explore new places and try new foods. But now he wants the same old thing every day. The other day I bought him new shoes. They were the kind with velcro fasteners that would have been so much easier to use. But he made such a fuss, I took them back. It just wasn't worth the bother. I exchanged them for some shoes just like his worn out ones and he was happy. - Norma Dupree

Norma gave up making things a little easier for her to make Jake happy. That was probably a good choice. However, sometimes a change that will make the caregiving job easier might be necessary.

The rule is to make *no unnecessary* changes and to make necessary ones in small increments while maintaining as much of the old as possible. If Norma had decided the shoes were necessary, she might have bought them in the same color and as close to the same style as Jake's old shoes. Then she'd have introduced them gradually by having Jake wear them an hour or so a day. Compliments about how good they looked on him would also help.

Routines, not adventures. Like variety and change, adventures tend to be fraught with hazards of the unknown. Routines give the patient a feeling of control because they know what will happen next. Develop a routine and try not to change it once it is set. Bedtime, mealtime, a weekly trip to a mall, a nightly TV show, all can be routines.

Emotions And Feelings Rule

Dementia-related behaviors are often driven by an emotion. And this emotion is often negative. A quick review of the chapters on emotions (Chapter 2) and thinking (Chapter 11) provides these highlights:

- ***Residual feelings.*** These are emotions held over from a past event.
- ***Negative feelings*** are strong, urgent and insistent and thus are usually the first ones noticed. Their job is to warn us of danger and push us into action.

- *Information plus emotion.* We naturally attach feelings to the events in our lives. The first one experienced is often a residual negative feeling demanding action now.
- *Vetting process.* The information with its attached feeling travels to the cognitive part of the brain where it is vetted--reviewed and judged for accuracy and appropriateness. If the initial feeling is deemed inaccurate, it is ignored.

The patient: With limited vetting skills, the patient's brain accepts the information and emotion as fact, often adding some drama to "make sense" of the situation.

- *Response vs. reaction.* We choose to respond, to decide to act or not act on the resulting information, emotions and drama, depending on a judgment of how helpful we believe that action will be.

The patient: With impaired ability to control impulses, the patient reacts to the first emotion they feel without attention to consequences.

The bottom line is that dementia keeps the patient from being in control of their actions, leaving them at the mercy of their emotions. Thus it becomes important to learn how to help the patient avoid those negative emotions that foster unwanted behaviors.

Comfort Is Key

Like security, comfort and any other positive feeling will serve to limit dementia-related behaviors. The patient may once have enjoyed a variety of challenging activities and viewed being a bit uncomfortable as a part of the deal. Not anymore. Comfort and feeling good is now the total goal.

Find ways to provide safety, comfort, peace, calmness, relaxation, happiness, enjoyment or almost any positive emotion and the behaviors will decrease. In fact, when a patient feels emotionally secure and physically comfortable, behaviors are less likely to occur at all and when they do, they will likely be less violent.

Here And Now Is All There Is

Place and time are concepts that no longer compute.

Only what the patient can see, hear or touch is real. The rest are concepts and take too much energy to compute, if it is possible at all.

We make sure someone visits Mom at least every other day, if not sooner. But Mom often greets me with, "Oh, honey, I'm so glad to see you. No one has been here for weeks! I put up a calendar and had all her visitors sign it but it didn't help. - Marion Peterson

The calendar has become another unfathomable concept. Mrs. Peterson lives in a world without past or future. Reminding her that Marion was there two days ago is useless. Yesterday is not accessible, nor is tomorrow. Mrs. Peterson would view "Wait a minute until I finish" as having to wait forever.

I want to go home. The exception to the here and now ideation is that emotional memory does last. Thus, "I want to go home" may actually mean "I want to *feel* the way I used to feel, before dementia, before I came here, before...."

24. Causes

triggers: Something that initiates a negative response in a patient.

environmental triggers: Those in the environment such as excesses, change or media.

physical triggers: Those that are body-related, such as illness or physical discomfort.

emotional triggers: Negative feelings, often generated by delusions but can also be anxiety from a variety of sources including environmental.

***

LBD-related behaviors can be LBD symptoms such as hallucinations and delusions themselves. However, actual behaviors are usually secondary. As verbal skills fail, behaviors become a person's major form of communication. Therefore, dementia-related behaviors are often reactions to:

- *LBD-related symptoms*. Examples: Accusations due to a delusion of a partner's infidelity or fright about a hallucination of wild animals in the house.
- *Environmental, physical or emotional discomfort.* Examples: Too many people talking at once, a UTI or frustration about their reality not being accepted.

LBD Symptoms

Some behaviors are actually symptoms of the disease:

Delusions show up when Lewy bodies cause thinking skills to fade. (See Chapter 7). These can be combined with hallucinations, real situations or information on the media, such as TV. There are also a wide variety of types of delusions. One is that of misidentification of a person or a place. When a person is involved this is called Capgras Syndrome, described earlier as a visual misperception. Another misidentification delusion, commonly called reduplicative paramnesia, involves places and locations.[51] Other common delusions involve infidelity, abandonment and theft.

Hallucinations show up when Lewy bodies are in the areas of the brain controlling vision and its perception. (See Chapter 17, Visual Symptoms). Hallucinations by themselves don't usually cause problems because the person understands that they aren't real. But then, the advancing disease compromises thinking skills and the person begins to believe their hallucinations are real and act accordingly.

Most hallucinations are benign and may bother the care partner more than the patient. If this is the case, they simply need to be accepted as a part of the patient's life. Occasionally hallucinations combine with past experiences such as war or a difficult childhood. Then the patient needs help to get rid of their scary and disturbing visions.

Moods. Depression, empathy deficit, anxiety and apathy can all be LBD related. See Chapter 20 for treatment of these disorders.

Other Triggers

Any environmental, physical or emotional discomfort can lead to dementia-related behaviors.

Environmental

Environmental issues involve maintaining comfort and keeping it simple. Change taxes a patient's cognitive skills. So does too much of almost anything. Even when these involve previously enjoyed activities, changes and excesses are likely to be burdensome.

Maintain the status-quo. Barbara Hutchinson and her husband Bill, who had advanced PDD, were masters at maintaining the status quo in a continually changing environment. They traveled for a year in their motor home, crossing the nation from Alaska to Florida, telling people about LBD and raising money for research.[52] Traveling, which involves continual change, is usually quite difficult for the LBD patient. Barb counteracted this by keeping the inside of their motor home a never changing environment where Bill could feel safe and comfortable. Bill tolerated and even enjoyed the trip.

Avoid excesses. With LBD, a person must focus on everything at once. They can't block out unwanted sounds or sights and focus on just one thing. Thus, an environment that is too busy can cause someone with

LBD to feel out of control and anxious. These feelings aren't easily verbalized, thus often show up as behaviors.

Too much noise, too much furniture or too many items on the furniture, too many people, too much going on at once, too much of almost anything including choices. Barb kept the clutter down in their motor home—no easy task in a small place! No matter where they were, Bill had the same easy chair, the same place at their table and the same bed. When life outside the motor home got too confusing and he started telegraphing his discomfort by acting confused and irritable, the Hutchinsons escaped to their familiar motor home sanctuary where Bill did not feel challenged beyond his ability to cope.

I read about the Hutchinsons. Their trip was so unbelievable. I can't imagine taking Mom on such an extended trip, even with a motor home! But I use Barb's environmental control ideas. I really limit the things in Mom's room. Mom's past the place where new clothes are exciting— anything new is more likely to be confusing! So even if I get something new for her, I try to make it as near like her old things as I can. And I don't keep all of it in her room at once. Just one or two dresses in her closet and only a few things in her drawers, for instance. All of this makes it much easier for Mom to choose what to wear and that always starts her day better. - Marion Peterson

Most of us couldn't do what Barbara and Bill did but we can learn from them and adapt their ideas to our patient's needs.

Develop routines. Once a routine is in place, it becomes automatic and requires very little thought. For the average person, this allows multitasking. For the patient, it allows them to continue doing activities they'd not be able to do otherwise and to feel a sense of control over their life.

Our days are the same, day in and day out. We eat at the same time and Jake naps at the same time and we watch the same TV shows in the evening. We even have routines around our shopping. We always go to the same stores and then to the same little restaurant for a snack. I'd love a little more variety but I know that the routine is important for Jake. - Norma Dupree

Norma can use Jake's nap time to give herself some variety. If she can feel comfortable leaving him alone, she can even go out for a visit with a friend.

Include tasks. Routines can include regular activities such as folding clothes. These help a patient feel useful and improve self-esteem.

Jake sets the table for every meal and when we are done, he takes the dirty dishes to the sink. When he has regular tasks to do, he's happier and acts out less." She smiles. "I could probably do the job better and more quickly myself, but seeing him happy and peaceful is well worth it. - Norma Dupree

Control media. Patients may perceive what they see on television or hear on the radio as real.

Peter's pretty weak and so it takes two of us to get him moved to his chair. The other evening, he was in his chair, watching a sitcom I didn't think would be too exciting. Was I wrong! I'd just stepped out of the room when I heard someone on TV yell 'Duck and dive' followed by an awful crash. I dashed back in the room and found Peter on the floor with his head half under the bed. - Jenny Ellis

As a child, Peter had lived in an area where earthquake drills taught children to duck and dive under their school desk. When he heard the earthquake warning in the sitcom, this super weak man perceived it as real and his body responded as it had been trained to do. Suddenly he had enough energy to bolt up out of his easy chair and try to dive under his bed.

His head was bleeding where he'd hit it on the leg of the bed, but otherwise, he seemed all right. His first words were, 'Was anyone else hurt?' - Jenny Ellis

Even after the fact, Mr. Ellis believed the earthquake was real. Not only does the LBD patient perceive the TV programs they watch as real, they often internalize them and incorporate them into their dreams, hallucinations or delusions.

Mom has been having delusions that she is being chased. I convinced her to change her TV viewing from her favorite cop shows to something less stimulating and the delusions stopped." (wry grin) Of course, every once in a while she manages to sneak in a cop show, especially

when we have new care staff. And then Mom has delusions for a while.
- Marion Peterson

When patients can't discriminate between media and real life, it is up to their caregivers and care staff to find ways to monitor their patient's viewing and eliminate shows that over-stimulate or install fear.

Physical

Poor communication skills. Due to the physical problems that accompany LBD and especially PDD, the LBD patient may lose communication skills early on, while his cognition is still fairly intact. The issue then is to find a way to communicate non-verbally.

Mom gets so frustrated when I don't understand what she's trying to tell me. Yesterday, she was asking for something--I still don't know what!-- and she got so mad she threw her spoon on the floor. - Marion Peterson

Mrs. Peterson substitutes odd words and mumbles so that she is often misunderstood, which frustrates her and leads to angry behaviors.

The behavior may also be the body's way of communicating pain or discomfort. Then the patient likely doesn't know what it is or possibly, even where it is. They just know that they hurt or are uncomfortable.

ANS malfunctions like constipation or urinary problems like UTIs often increase acting-out behavior. In fact, caregivers soon learn that unusual acting out can signal a urinary infection even before there are any other signs of infection.

When Jake starts having more hallucinations than normal or becomes overly anxious, I've learned to test his urine. Usually, I'll find an infection. As soon I get it treated, Jake starts acting more normal. - Norma Dupree

Hidden injuries. If you can find no ANS dysfunctions, check for hidden injuries. The patient may not be able to communicate well enough to let you know—or sometimes, even to know themselves!— that there is something wrong. In her classic article on behavior management and dementia, Dr. Tanis Ferman[53] tells of a patient who happily swept floors all day. When he stopped and became combative, the staff looked for the usual problems without success. He didn't have

139

a urinary infection, constipation or a change in routine. Then a physical examination exposed a broken thumb. They fixed that and the man peacefully went back to his sweeping.

Emotional

Emotions drive most behaviors. (See Chapter 2).

Jake's behavior gets worse when he's anxious, like when we go to the mall and there's a lot of people around. He gets frustrated more easily then and that quickly turns to anger, especially when I can't understand what he's trying to tell me. It doesn't have to be anything important, just some simple thing and he's furious. - Norma Dupree

Yes, emotions rule! In addition, any naturally occurring negative feeling is likely to be exaggerated and foster unwanted behaviors. It's normal to feel frustrated when you can't get your message across but Jake has only "angry" and "not angry." He can't control intensity and so Norma gets the full blast every time.

25. Behavior Management

non-disruptive behaviors: Those behaviors that may distress the care partner but do not distress the patient.

empathy: Being able to put yourself in another's shoes.

acceptance: Accepting another person's reality without necessarily believing it.

speak to the emotion: Voice the emotion being expressed by the patient.

distraction: Something that draws the patient's attention away from the present behavior.

bribe: An inducement to stop whatever the patient is doing.

listening: A more successful response than explaining.

apologizing: A great tool for deflecting anger.

***

Non-Disruptive Behaviors

Often, behaviors such as hallucinations or mild delusions do not bother the patient. However, if the care partner or staff tries to use reason to explain or change the behavior, this futile effort will likely leave the patient emotionally upset and feeling unheard. Then their previously benign behavior is likely to become disruptive!

Hallucinations are what triggered us into taking Hilda to a doctor to see what was wrong. She kept seeing things I couldn't see. She wasn't scared but she sure was upset that I couldn't see them. They were so clear to her! - Barney Darnell

It wasn't the hallucination but Hilda's perceived lack of support from her husband that led to her disruptive behavior.

Help care partners to let go of such efforts and simply accept this behavior as a part of the disease. "It's not my loved one, it is the disease.

Empathy And Acceptance

The patient experiences the reason for their behavior as unchangeable fact, their only truth. They can't change. Only you can change the way you respond to their behaviors. Being empathetic helps you to do this.

Try this experiment in empathy: Think about how you'd feel if someone told you that something you held to be unalterably true was not and then did their best to convince you of their way of thinking. What negative feelings come up when they won't accept what you say? When they patiently explain away what you know is true? Or impatiently argue? Do you feel unheard, angry or hurt? Do you feel isolated or unloved? Do you feel insulted or belittled? (Only your initial reaction counts, since it is the one the person living with LBD is stuck with.)

Now imagine this: You again tell your companion about something that you know without a doubt that they did to hurt you. They cry and defend themselves against your obviously correct assertions. What are your initial reactions now? Are they similar to those above?

These are all feelings that come up for the patient whose reasons for their behaviors are not accepted.

The care partner or staff who doesn't accept adds a wall of negative feelings to the experience similar to that in the experiment above. The patient sees explaining as belittling; arguing as unwillingness to listen and defending as flat-out lying. When you let go of your need to be right and accept the patient's reality as the only one they have, the negative feelings and their accompanying behaviors decrease.

Try this experiment in acceptance: Imagine the same scene as above but your companion accepts what you say at face value. They smile, nod and maybe ask a question. What were your feelings now? Validation? Acceptance? Other positive feelings? Did your anxiety go down?

Now imagine this: Imagine that you make the same accusations with the same firmness of belief. This time they don't argue. Instead they apologize. Was it harder to continue being angry even though you had every right to be? How did the apology feel? (First feeling only, remember, that's all that counts. The second feeling of, "sure, but they don't mean it" comes from your complex thinking.)

Acceptance is not the same as believing. It is allowing a person to have their own reality without trying to change it. When a child invites you to a make-believe tea party, you join in their reality. You play along but you don't really believe there is any tea in your cup. In this same way, you can join a patient's reality.

Join the patients in their reality. Do not try to convince them that what they see or believe isn't real. If you consider that a person with LBD is by definition, incapable of reasoning, insisting on rational thinking doesn't make sense. You have to meet the patient where they are. Think of this as their reality. Once you are communicating on the same level, you can gently guide them back to *your* reality.

Jake used to see children coming out from behind the television set. I'd go look and say something like, "Come on kids, time to go home." Then I'd usher them out the door. - Norma Dupree

When Norma joined Jake in his reality, she was able to move the action in a direction to where it was no longer a problem for him or for her.

When Jenny Ellis found that her husband was convinced that one of his nursing home caregivers was "bad," she knew that it would do no good to try to change his mind, even though there was no evidence that this aide had ever been anything but nice to Mr. Ellis. Jenny simply asked that a different aide be assigned to him until he "forgot." She knew that it would do no good to try to reason with him but she also knew that his delusions tended to disappear eventually if he was not reminded of them.

Peter was convinced that Joan, one of his nursing aides, wanted to hurt him. By now, I knew enough not to try to convince him otherwise. Instead I apologized to him for his hurt. Then I asked the nurse to assign him a different aide until he "forgot." A couple of weeks later, Joan was again assigned to Peter. He didn't have a problem with her at all...he'd forgotten all about his fears, thank goodness. - Jenny Ellis

They were fortunate. Peter might have remembered--emotional memories can last a long time.

Don't explain: listen. Explaining away the patient's only reality fosters feelings of insult and belittlement. Listen and the patient will feel heard.

Don't argue: accept. Arguing feels like rejection and fosters more angry behavior. Accept and the patient will feel validated.

Don't defend: apologize. Defending feels like downright lies. An apology will deflect the patient's anger. (Yes, let go of having to be right and just go ahead and apologize!)

Jenny listened, accepted her husband's reality, apologized and did what she could to decrease his worry by asking to have Joan's assignment changed.

Don't take the behavior personally. Accepting the behavior does not mean that you accept responsibility for it. The care person's mantra needs to be "It is the disease not the person." The disease and its symptoms drive the patient to believe and act the way they do.

When Jake accused me of wanting to run away with some other man, I was shocked and hurt. I've never given him a reason not to trust me and at one time he knew that. But then I started telling myself over and over, "It's the disease talking, not my husband." - Norma Dupree

Care partners say they have to do this daily, sometimes minute by minute. It is not easy to deal with anger, combativeness and other acting-out behaviors that appear for no apparent reason.

Speak To The Emotion

Speaking to an emotion can often do wonders at deflecting anger, fear or other negative feelings, thus changing the behavior.

Jake got combative in the ER when I told him I'd put him on the waiting list for a bed in Anytown. - Norma Dupree

It was an easy guess that Jake was experiencing a fear of abandonment.

I tried to explain to Jake that even if he was in a care facility, I'd be there for him but that just made him worse. - Norma Dupree

Since for Jake, there is no past or future, a fear that something *might happen* means that it *is happening*. Thus to Jake, Norma's explanations are obviously lies...In his reality, she has already abandoned him.

144

His rejection really hurt but I stopped trying to explain. Instead, I told him, "It must really hurt to think I'd leave you." He took a deep breath and nodded but he still acted angry with me. I followed that up too: "You must be really angry right now." He nodded and even smiled a little. - Norma Dupree

When Norma accepted Jake's reality, he felt heard and he began to be able to hear Norma. When she spoke to his fear, he began to feel understood and was able to start relaxing. This process holds true for any of the patient's expressed emotions, not just fear of abandonment. When a patient feels heard and supported, the need for behavior decreases greatly.

Then I added in a firm voice, "Well, I'm right here and I won't let anything bad happen to you." - Norma Dupree

Take sides. Be the champion, the rescuer. Once Jake was calmer, Norma took on a strong, supportive attitude and told him she was there for him, on his side. This might not work with someone who could think of the future but again, Jake lives in the here and now.

Voice first. Norma didn't try to touch Jake until he was completely over his angry outburst. To do so would be to trigger his defensiveness and invite the behavior to return, perhaps even more violently.

Use touch. Touching has been shown to be a very effective mode of communication with dementia patients.[54] Using a gentle voice and giving a hug or a kind touch will go far towards calming down a dementia patient.

Use Distractions And Bribes

Once a patient has begun to calm down, distraction will move them away from an uncomfortable issue.

When Jake had calmed down, I asked him if he'd like to go have some ice cream. (Smile) That usually works. Jake does like his ice cream! - Norma Dupree

Jake's short attention span along with his difficulty focusing makes distraction a useful tool. However, it wouldn't have worked if Norma had tried to use it while Jake was walled off by his negative emotions.

However, once the anger has been deflected, Norma's bribe of ice cream worked like a charm.

Bribes are great tools for dementia patients. Unlike children, who can learn to manipulate when bribed, these patients simply respond to a pleasant experience in the here and now. Then, once their attention is on the bribe, the earlier behavior is forgotten.

Distractions are a mixed blessing however. They can also interfere with a conversation. If you want to get your patient's attention, decrease distractions.

If I want to be sure David hears me, I've found that I have the best success when I'm standing in front of him in a quiet room. Touching helped as well, especially when I want to make a point." Marie Newman: "

Marie has learned how to limit distractions so that she can get her message across as easily as possible. She has also learned the power of touch.

Be Positive

While negative emotions are the ones that demand attention, positive ones are what keeps a person healthy.

Offer ongoing positive attention. Ongoing gentle, non-custodial touching and caring verbal messages helps a patient feel more emotionally secure and less vulnerable to the fear of abandonment. The more loved and valued a person feels, the fewer behaviors we see.

I've started hugging Jake a lot more than I used to. And I'm telling him all the time how much I love him and appreciate him and need him. It hasn't stopped his accusations altogether, but they aren't as common now. - Norma Dupree

Jake probably doesn't remember Norma's actions or her words but with his emotional memory still intact, he does remember the emotions involved and they provide a cushion of safety for him.

Make copious use of compliments. Norma can also expound generously and continually about how she feels as long as her actions match her words. Jake's thinking abilities can't discriminate enough to pick up exaggeration but he does pay attention to actions before words.

Keep It Simple.

When the patient has only one or two things to focus on, they can feel safe and functional. Add more and they will begin to feel overpowered and anxious...negative feelings that can lead to a meltdown. Avoid excesses of any kind:

Eliminate clutter. Clutter is confusing to a person who has difficulty focusing on one thing at a time.

Avoid crowds. Visit malls at slow times. Invite no more than two friends to visit at a time--and remind them to talk only one at a time.

Avoid loud noises and bright lights. LBD often increases sensitivities in other areas than drugs. Keep sunglasses handy and use them freely, even inside.

Limit choices to no more than two. "Do you want this blouse or this one?" Not "Which of these blouses in your closet do you want?"

Even when certain tasks get too difficult, a patient can still do them with help.

Use patience. This is true for everything involving a dementia patient but especially true when helping them to perform a task. What used to be second nature now may need to be processed slowly before it can be turned into action.

Use steps. Break larger tasks into a series of smaller steps. Gently remind them of steps they forget and help them with the ones they can no longer do. Visual cues like signs or examples help too.

Marion: "Every morning Mom and I brush her teeth. She does the work, I'm along as coach. I tell her how, each step at a time and sometimes I have to show her. I have to remember not to get too far ahead because then I'm giving her too many choices. She gets confused and says, 'Oh, dear, I don't know...I just don't know...' and stops doing anything."

Working with an LBD patient is like the AA slogan, you know the one that says, 'One step at a time." If you get too far ahead you lose them!

Be a model. We all pick up on behaviors before we do words. A person's first reaction to a behavior is to react in kind. Thus, if you show anger, impatience or any negative emotion, the patient will automatically react negatively. However, you can break this cycle because you don't have to react to their negative behaviors; you can make a conscious choice to respond positively. When you respond calmly and positively, you provide a model for the patient. This makes it easier for them to let go of their emotion-driven behaviors.

I've learned to listen calmly to David's tirades, then nod and smile. Usually, he'll calm down then and I can suggest some distraction like watching TV. - Marie Newman

Marie has learned not to respond to a negative with another negative. That only makes the situation worse. Instead she accepts calmly, which deflects his anger instead of reflecting it.

Medical Management

Dementia experts recommend that non-drug options be tried first before resorting to behavior management drugs. However, these drugs usually become, if not necessary, then very useful before the dementia journey is over.

Dementia Drugs.

Dementia drugs tend to decrease all dementia symptoms including dementia-related behaviors, especially when used with a variety of non-medical methods for behavior management. These should be the first drugs considered. Eventually, other medication may be necessary. (See Chapter 12, Dementia Drugs.)

Antipsychotic Drugs

Once all non-drug options for behavior management have been considered and tried, physicians may prescribe one of the second-generation, atypical antipsychotics such as Seroquel. These drugs must be given "off label" but can often be helpful. Equally often they can cause serious sensitivity issues and so they should be monitored carefully.

Nuplazid is an atypical antipsychotic with a different action than the earlier atypicals and is supposed to cause fewer sensitivity issues. However, it is quite expensive. It is approved for use with Parkinson's with psychosis but regularly used off-label for both types of LBD as well. When "Parkinson's with psychosis" becomes "Parkinson's with dementia" seems somewhat cloudy. For example, Nuplazid is approved for treatment of delusions, which are evidence of a loss of thinking ability, which in turn, indicates at least mild cognitive impairment (MCI), if not dementia.

Behavior management drugs can provide a quick result and are therefore especially useful during a crisis situation, where the patient is out of control and/or acting violently. Once they are calmed down, other options can be tried. (See more in Chapter 16, Drug Sensitivity.)

Medical Marijuana

Most states have now legalized medical marijuana. Even if the patient lives in a state where it is not yet legal, it can be obtained easily via the internet. Until recently, it like most herbal treatments, had many antidotal claims for pain management unsupported by any clinical trials. However, this may change soon. As of 2018, clinical trials were in process.[55] In the meantime, many care partners say that it has provided pain control for both their loved ones and themselves, with fewer side effects than prescribed drugs like opiates or over-the-counter drugs such as aspirin.[56] When a patient's pain decreases, decreased behavior usually follows. And a care partner with less pain will usually be less stressed and this decreased stress will be modeled by their loved one.

Medical marijuana may also be useful for treating symptoms such as hallucinations. While THC (tetrahydrocannabinol) is the psychoactive part of the cannabis plant, CBD (cannabidiol) is a natural antipsychotic that balances THC's hallucinogenic effects. Used alone, it seems to reduce the amount of brain activity that causes psychotic symptoms, with far fewer side effects than other antipsychotics.

CBD usually comes in an oil that can be administered via vaping, as a tincture, with topical solutions or in capsule or gummy drop forms. Vaping and tincture drops under the tongue will enter the blood stream quickly. Capsules and gummy drops must be digested, which takes more time and makes them less potent. Topical solutions of CBD oil mixed with a lubricant such as coconut oil allows you to target a specific area.

149

The down side of CBD use is that it is seldom if ever recognized by insurance companies and tends to be expensive, especially compared to OTC drugs or insurance-covered drugs with a low co-pay. Also, like all herbal treatments, it is mostly unrecognized by the FDA, and therefore, uncontrolled. You must depend on the authenticity of the seller and manufacturer to get what you are buying.

Combining Drugs With Non-Drug Options

Additional medication does not preclude the use of good behavior-management techniques. In fact, it may be the other way around. The continued or additional use of these options along with the drugs often results in smaller drug doses for equally good or even better outcomes. This is especially important as drug sensitivity is often connected to the size of the dose.

One advantage of combined use is that while the dosage may be smaller, the wanted result usually occurs more quickly.

Short Term Use

It can be helpful to consider a short term course of mild antipsychotics to assist with additional stress that major changes such as a move from home to a care center can cause.

We've finally got Peter's Seroquel level to where it helps him without making things worse. And so when Peter's doctor suggested we increase his dosage when we moved Peter into residential treatment, I was against it. I didn't want to mess with what was working! But the doctor explained that it would be temporary, just long enough to help him settle in. -- Jenny Ellis

The doctor started Peter's the additional mild antipsychotic a week prior to his move, since it takes a while for the drug to work. He decreased it three weeks later, when Peter was beginning to feel comfortable in his new room.

These drugs may also be helpful in a crisis, where the patient is out of control and especially when they are violent. Once they are calmed down, other options can be tried. Of course, if care partner and staff act with empathy and acceptance quickly, many crises--but not all--can be averted.

150

Support

Caring for the LBD patient takes a team. The care professionals, the care partners and even the patients have their own tasks. However, to do a good job, you all need to act as a team, with support for each other. Ideally, all of you will have done your homework and will be knowledgeable about LBD. Each of you needs to recognize the other's strengths—and where you personally most need support and help. When you work together, you will find that your special skills will combine with those of others on the team to provide the patient with the best care possible.

But it is important to know about what each group needs as well. For example, you need to have access to good education about the disease and all the care partners can teach you about their loved ones. The care partners and families need encouragement for good self-care and all the special information you can teach them about the disease and how to deal with it safely. And finally, the patient needs to feel as independent as possible while still receiving the physical care they need.

And finally, we all need support as we deal with end of life issues. Thankfully, hospice services are there to help. This service doesn't have to wait until the end is very near. Hospice is for the living, not the dying! It is for helping patients and their families live through the last months of the patient's life in ways as fulfilling, gentle and caring as possible.

26. Support for the Care Professional

The goals of care staff and care partner are similar: a well-cared-for patient. Both need support to be able to do that well. Many times this support overlaps. Supporting the care staff supports the care partner and supporting the care partner supports the patient.

LBD Specific Education

You don't need degrees or years of training but you do need to educate yourself about Lewy body diseases and Lewy body dementia in particular. You are already on your way if you're reading this book.

- *Other books and articles about LBD.* Find a list of our choices in Resources.
- *LBDA.org website.* Find a wealth of information here.
- *LBD online Caregiver support groups.* There are several that you can visit even if you aren't a care partner. They give you an inside view about issues like medications and behaviors and about the everyday life of an LBD care partner. Find a list of these in Resources.
- *In-house training.* Ask that the dementia care training provided by your facility include information about LBD and its drug sensitivities specifically.

LBD Library

It helps to have informational resources handy at work for quick reference when computers are not available. If your workplace already has a library, ask them to provide an LBD section. Add such items as:

- *Downloaded copies of articles* posted on the LBDA website or other sources. Include articles on:
  - o LBD, PDD and DLB.
  - o Caregiving and the dementia patient.
  - o Behavior management.
  - o Hospice and LBD.

- *Books on LBD* and dementia care. Care partners are often glad to donate these to any group that shows an interest.
- *DVDs* on LBD and dementia such as Teepa Snow's Lewy Body Dementia: What Everyone Needs to Know, available on Amazon.
- *A list of YouTube and other online aids.* Those on the resource list on Pines Education Institute's Dementia Care Academy, can be viewed over and over, alone or in groups.[57]
- *A list of relevant websites, articles and books* so that care staff can do further research.

Behavior Management

Using behavior management skills with a dementia patient makes your job easier and less frustrating--and your patient happier.

Books on behavior management. Include our book, *Responsive Dementia Care: Fewer Behaviors Fewer Drugs,* as well as some of the books and articles recommended in that book.

Behavior management training. This is different from LBD specific education although there will be many crossovers. Ask that it include specifically acceptance, empathy and dementia-related communication skills. It should include an experiential segment, where you can experience how the patient feels.

Practice these skills until they become second-nature for you.

Supervisor Training. For you to give your best service, your supervisors need to be educated about LBD too. For example, they need to know about LBD's:

- *Slowness,* so that they will allow adequate time for good patient care when they assign patients to you.
- *Fluctuations.* They should know that LB patients will show different levels of ability and awareness at different times—and that the patients aren't faking when they appear more or less confused than they did at another time.
- *Acting-out behaviors* of LBD so they can provide additional help, guidance and medication as needed.

- *Medication and drug sensitivity issues* so that when you report changes they can interpret them properly and notify the physician if needed.

Before we put Mom into Anytown Center, I talked to the Director of Nurses. We agreed on a schedule that worked for Mom and fit with the facility's schedule. Mom couldn't have everything the same but I knew going in that she'd have the important things, like the medications that she needs at times when they worked best for her. I made sure I could still help with Mom's care. The Director explained that there were certain things that I couldn't do because of insurance—like lifting her on and off the commode. She told me that the aides would welcome my help in other ways like helping her bathe, get dressed or taking her out to eat in her wheelchair. Knowing ahead of time what I could and couldn't do saved me a lot of frustration later on. And having the aides know at the beginning that I expected to be a part of the treatment team helped too. We really are a team! - Marion Peterson

By recruiting the director before placement and making sure the director knew her mother's special needs, Marion felt herself to be a part of the care team from the start. With the guidance from the director, the care providers also knew what to expect from Marion and worked with her from the beginning.

Safety

Safe work habits keep both you and your patient safe. Here are some suggestions specific to your safety:

- *Use proper lifting techniques.* Keep your gait belt handy and use it to keep both you and the patient safe.
- *Know what to do when a patient unexpectedly turns violent.* In the home, the caregiver probably can tell you what works best for their loved one. If you work in a facility that doesn't have a safety plan, ask for one.
- *Ask for help.* If you have any doubts about being able to do a job by yourself, ask a co-worker for help. Remember that an LBD patient may be quite able to help himself today and almost helpless tomorrow—or vise versa.

Self-Care

A healthy and happy care person usually has a more contented, easier-to-handle patient.

- *Cultivate a healthy life style* with plenty of exercise and good diet so you can do the physical tasks better and more easily.
- *Maintain a positive attitude.* Your attitude will be reflected by your patients.
- *Maintain outside interests, hobbies and friends.* Have a life away from your job. This helps you to be objective and to see a patient's needs separate from your own needs.

27. Support for the Care Partner

The care partner is the most important person in a patient's life, their lifeline, their connection to continuity and the person who knows them best. The care partner seldom chooses this job, any more than their loved one chooses their illness.[c]

I didn't sign on for this. It was not the way I planned to spend my retirement years. But I love my husband and I want to be here for him. - Jenny Ellis

A care partner is usually someone who, once the need is there, steps up and does the job with love to the best of her ability.

My mother-in-law gave me a lot, especially after my husband died. Now it is my turn to give to Mom. Neither of us planned it this way but I'm glad I'm here and able to help. - Marion Peterson

Care Partner Issues

Care partners often deal with personal issues like these:

Guilt. Most care partners will have some guilt about placing their loved one in a care facility. Many spousal care partners are elderly with health problems of their own. Younger care partners are often adult children with conflicting responsibilities such as families or work that make home care difficult or even unsafe. When these problems lead to a care partner's inability to care for her loved one without help, she may feel that she has failed. Feelings of inadequacy and guilt may drive her to be critical and demanding with you as a way to feel as though they are helping their loved one.

Poor self-care. By the time you come into the picture, a care partner has usually become so invested in caring for her loved one that everything else has gone by the wayside. She is so focused on her job that she forgets to care for herself. She has put off her friends so often

---

[c] **Reminder:** About three-fourths all LBD care partners are female. Thus in this section, we use feminine pronouns. This does not discount male care partners like author James but is simply for easier reading.

they've stopped calling. She has given up activities she once enjoyed because it is just too difficult to get away. She neglects to see her dentist, puts off going to her doctor and seldom sees a hairdresser. When she does go out, she hurries back.

Inadequate sleep. Care partners often complain that they don't get enough sleep. Their loved one's Active Dreams and other night time behaviors have often deprived a care partner of sleep. Sometimes a care partner is afraid to sleep soundly for fear her loved one will need her and she won't hear.

Increased responsibility. A care partner takes on more and more responsibility as her loved one's condition degenerates. Often this is responsibility that once was shared or even carried mainly by the patient. The care partner seldom wants this but now she feels stuck with it.

Jake used to pay all our bills but he got to where he couldn't concentrate and so I took it over. Now he has become fanatical about my 'spending too much.' He questions me about everything I buy. I understand it is Jake's way of trying to maintain control but I still feel frustrated. (sigh) It's the disease, not my husband. It's the disease, not my husband. It's the... - Norma Dupree

Norma is expressing pain and frustration of unwanted responsibility-- and her loved one's difficulty in giving up tasks that he felt defined him as an adult.

Care partners also have problems giving up responsibility for their loved one once they've taken it on.

More than anything I miss the partner I used to have. Peter was my best friend. We did everything together. Now I have to make the decisions and telling him my troubles just makes him upset. He isn't able to support me anymore. (shakes her head) I thought I'd be glad to give up some of that responsibility. I certainly didn't want it all in the first place! But now, I find myself second-guessing the care staff, trying to tell them their job. - Jenny Ellis

Like Jake, Jenny is trying to maintain control, to hang on to the job that defined her for years and now, keeps her connected to her husband in a time of change.

Providing Support

The fact that the care partner is so important to your patient makes the care partner equally important to you. The patient tends to reflect the feeling of their care partner. Thus, unless you have the support of your patient's care partner, you will have a resistant patient. You will work harder with a less happy result. The way you get support from a care partner is by first supporting her.

Listen with respect. A care partner usually knows her patient's responses to his disease better than anyone else. Over the years, she's learned what he likes and what he doesn't. Through trial and error, she's learned what works and what doesn't. Show gratitude for this and use it to make both the patient's life and yours easier.

Use her knowledge and add to it. She has probably read everything she could find about LBD. Believe the care partner when she tells you that LBD is different from other dementias. Do your homework so you will understand what she is talking about. Although you may know what to expect with Alzheimer's, there are differences with each LBD patient. Reading this book and others about LBD will help but the care partner will still be the expert on her patient. Listen to her and respect what she says.

Be a co-worker. You and the care partner are co-workers with the patient's comfort as your mutual goal. You provide the physical help and safety the care partner can no longer provide. The care partner's jobs are that of patient advocate, provider of emotional support and the person who knows the patient best. Convince her that no one else can do these jobs as well as she can. The resulting increased sense of value will make it easier for her to let go of her guilt at "deserting" her loved one to the care of others.

I shudder to think how bossy I was when Peter was first put into the dementia care wing. I had to tell the aide everything. I didn't like the way they made the bed. I hated how the meals were served. Now I've learned to let them do their job and focus only on the ways I can help Peter. When I began to see the care providers as part of our team instead of opponents, Peter started getting much better care! And the care provider was more willing to listen to me when I said that Peter would take his meds better with pudding than applesauce. He doesn't like apples but he loves chocolate! - Jenny Ellis

Jenny and Peter Ellis had been doing well by themselves until his surgery. Jenny resented that this couldn't continue and the care providers took the brunt of her unconscious anger at her loss of control. The care staff shrugged off Jenny's irritability with sympathetic smiles. They listened to her suggestions and acted on them. When Jenny began to see that she still had value, she became less adversarial.

Be a friend. Take some time to visit with the care partner. This will often lift her spirits and what helps her, helps the patient. This is not just idle chatting although it can and should be enjoyable. It is actually therapeutic for both care partner and the patient. Over time, a care partner's outside contacts dwindle, with few social contacts save for those she meets in doctor's offices and shopping.

Thank goodness for our home health aide! She gives me a chance to escape the house, even if it is just to go shopping. I used to be able to run out and do an hour's shopping or even go visit with a friend but I can't leave Jake alone anymore. It just isn't safe. The health aide and I have become good friends too and that helps even when I don't leave. - Norma Dupree

In a facility, help the care partner to feel at home. Show her where the coffee is and have a refrigerator for snacks that she can "raid." Spend some time visiting, asking about her family, her life away from the facility. You may feel rushed, as though you already have more than you can do but you will recoup the time you spend by having a more cooperative patient.

Do your job well. The care partner needs to see that you know your job. She needs to see, among other things, that you know how to lift, that you know behavior management techniques and that you enjoy what you are doing. Given this, she can feel more comfortable leaving her loved one with you. If not, she will have difficulty trusting her loved one to your care and may try to direct your every move!

Encourage Self-care. Once you have a care partner's trust, you can begin encouraging her to take care of herself. Encourage her to:

- *Take some "me time,"* like shopping, a lunch with a friend, a movie.
- *Get enough sleep.* You can suggest she take a nap while you are there if she appears tired.
- *Do some personal things* like getting her hair done. An improved appearance goes a long way towards improving self-image.
- *Keep her doctor and dental appointments.* She may have let these slide.

Remind her that she is a valuable part of her loved one's care and as such, she needs to take care of herself so that she can do her job. This is a very true statement. There is no one as lonely as a dementia patient whose care partner has passed away.

Encourage support groups. Care partners have usually been isolated in their homes with only their loved one for company. Once a care partner learns to trust you and sees you as a co-worker and friend, she can share with you. But you go home at night. You have a life separate from your job. For a care partner, her job IS her life, at least for now. A support group provides a forum where she can share her thoughts and feelings with people who relate because they've been or are where she is.

Thank goodness I have my group. When my health aide insisted that I go to a support group, I wasn't sure I should leave Jake that long. But I come back feeling so much better and more able to cope. They can relate. I hate to bore my friends with my ups and downs and besides, they don't really understand. My family supports me but they don't understand either. You can't if you haven't lived it. And Jake's sons...well...I'm grateful they understand better than they did before they talked to Jake's doctor, but they still have a long way to go. - Norma Dupree

Norma's group relates because they have the same issues she does. She can vent and her group knows she is simply frustrated, she doesn't want out. She can ask, "How do you handle this?" and get answers from others who have had the same problem. She can joke about her situation and her group will laugh with her. She goes home feeling better about herself and her situation. Here are some ways you can help care partners find a group:

- You can find a list of local LBD support groups on the LBDA website.[58]
- If there isn't a LBD group in your community, look for groups that might be supportive of a LBD care partner. A good source for finding other groups is the Family Caregiver Alliance.[59] You can go to this online site and find a variety of resources in your state.
- The Alzheimer's Association and various Parkinson's organizations will likely offer groups in your area.

Alzheimer's groups can provide support for dementia problems but may find LBD's unique symptoms like hallucinations and Active Dreams out of their ken. PD groups are great for movement issues but since patients often attend these groups with their care partners, the dementia symptoms tend to be avoided. If a group cannot support a care partner adequately, it only increases their sense of isolation. A good LBD support group will:

- Have a facilitator who is familiar with both DLB and PDD.
- Have at least two other group members whose loved ones have LBD.
- Exclude patients for at least some of the meetings. (This is a care partner choice but most LBD care partners prefer the freedom of discussing their loved ones dementia and acting-out issues without the patient present.)
- Keep a LBD Information File and Library. If the meeting is held in a care facility, this may be the same library that is available for professionals.
- Be a good resource for the location and value of other resources such as virtual and other local support groups, hospices and senior service organizations as well as local doctors, care facilities, day care centers and other services.
- Be a referral source of local LBD specialists, including neurologists, family physicians, occupational and voice therapists, dieticians, social workers and more.

Encourage adult day care.[60] This serves as a social outlet for the patient who still lives at home and as a few hours of respite for the care partner. It can also be a first step towards entry into a care facility.

28. Support for the Patient

If the patient's care partner has accepted you and is working well with you, the patient probably will too. A competent professional with a genuine liking for the elderly and for their job in general will usually have no problem developing the rapport and trust one needs to be able to support the patient. Supporting the patient involves:

Know the disease. Do your homework. Include:

- The education mentioned in Chapter 25.
- The patient specific information you learn from the care partner.

Respect the patient. Show this by:

- Giving him[d] the benefit of the doubt concerning his cognitive abilities. Limited communication skills may make it easy for you to assume your patient has fewer cognitive abilities than he does.
- Chatting with the patient and giving him time to answer, even if it is only the nod of a head.
- Not talking down or treating him like a child. He may have diminished capabilities but he is still an adult and wants to be treated as such.

Time And Communication

Everything goes slower for the LBD patient. Thinking, doing and especially communicating. If rushed, a patient will likely withdraw or become agitated. Give the patient the time he needs by:

- Practicing patience with everything you do with a LBD patient. Relax. If you feel rushed, the patient will too and will become more confused and less able to help with their own care.
- Counting to 10--or better yet, 30 (to yourself, please!) after you ask a question.

---

[d] **Reminder**: Since at least 60% of LBD patients are men, we use masculine pronouns in this section for easier reading. This is not to discount the many female patients such as Mrs. Peterson.

- Asking questions with no more than two clear choices. "Do you want to wear the red blouse or the white blouse?" is better (and quicker) than "Which blouse do you want to wear?"
- Asking questions with yes-no answers. (Two clear choices)
- Avoiding open ended questions that will confuse the patient and stop their communication.

Abandonment Issues

If the care partner has been reluctant or unable to include anyone else in the care of their loved one, strong dependence often develops on the patient's part.

This patient will respond with unwelcome behaviors when his care partner leaves him with anyone else. The result is often a care partner who is even more reluctant to leave.

- Utilize the patient's Good Times to discuss changes and introduce new people.
- If the care partner can consult with the patient about the change during their "Good Times," it seems to reduce agitation even if the patient doesn't remember later.
- Arrange to be with the patient and care partner together several times before she leaves him alone with you.
- Find a way to connect with the patient, some hobby or interest that you can share.

Control

A dementia patient is continually struggling to maintain control as he gradually loses the ability to do things he once took for granted.

- ***Include him.*** Tell him what you are planning to do before you do it thus making him part of the process.
- ***Encourage self-help.*** Encourage him to do everything he can for himself, even if it would be easier for you to do it. Let him wash his own face, feed himself, reach for his own coffee. So what if he doesn't do as well as you would? So what if he spills a bit? So what if it takes twice as long? The more you can allow a LBD patient to do things for himself, the more likely you will have a

happy, better functioning patient. In the long run, it will take you less time to give better care.

- ***Give him clear choices.*** "Do you want this robe around you?" not, "Which robe do you want around you?"

Unwanted Behaviors

Dementia patients impulsively act out whatever they are feeling. LBD patients take this one step further. Vivid hallucinations and organized delusions can populate the LBD patient's reality and increase what appears to be irrational behavior.

- With the LBD patient's drug sensitivity issues in mind, all care staff and care partners need to know and use non-medical techniques whenever possible. (See Chapter 25).
- Ask the care partner which techniques worked best for them.
- If the patient develops delusions about you, don't try to reason them away. You may have to change duties with another staff person for the time that the delusion lasts—usually no longer than a few days or weeks. When the patient has "forgotten" the delusion, you will probably be able to work with him again.

Fluctuating Cognition

By the time you see an LBD patient, Bad Times will likely be the norm. But there will still be the occasional moments of clarity. (Review Chapter 14)

- ***Learn the patient's cognitive schedule***—if there is one. When is he most likely to be alert? For how long?
- ***Use times of clarity.*** Learn from the care partner when clarity is most likely and how to best to use it. Don't assume the patient is faking when they fall back into confusion.
- ***Be alert for change.*** The patient's cognitive level can change quickly. You want to provide your LBD patients with as much freedom as they can handle. Still, you don't want them to fall because they've suddenly forgotten what they can and cannot do.
- ***Use a gait belt*** as a normal part of the patient's clothing. This gives you a quick way to grab hold if he suddenly becomes unstable.

I waited until Hilda was having a good day to tell her we needed to move into the Care Center. She was able to discuss it with me and agreed that I needed more help than she could give me. Although Hilda didn't remember our discussion, she accepted the move better than she did when I made changes without her input. - Barney Darnell

Care partners say that even if their loved one doesn't remember being consulted, they aren't as concerned about the change later. Also they both appreciate that small taste of what used to be normal as they make the decision together. As Barney did, you too can make use of the patient's good times to help them feel more in control of their care.

Documentation

As one of the people who have the most contact with the patient, your observations are valuable. Your careful nursing notes should include such items as these and more:

- The services you provided.
- The patient's level of cognition.
- The patient's mood....are they depressed, apathetic, happy?
- Any ongoing physical challenges, bruises, injuries or infections.
- Any evidence of new physical challenges such as redness on areas susceptible to bedsores or signs of a UTI.
- The patient's behavior: is it cooperative, resistant or apathetic. Is the behavior normal for that patient or is it a change? How?
- Any changes in behavior or any physical changes.
- Visitors and the patient's response to them.
- Reactions that may have been due to medication, especially a new prescription.

Medications

You may not be qualified to administer the patient's medication but you still need to know the following for anyone whose care is in your charge:

- What the patient is taking.
- Why he is taking it.
- What its expected result should be.
- What are the possible side effects.

- Drug issues specific to the patient's diagnosis. For example, with LBD, medications given for cognition can affect motor function and medications given for behavior or motor dysfunctions can affect cognition.

If you are a hands-on care person, you are the one most directly involved with the patient besides the care partner. As such, you will often to be the first person to see behavior or cognition changes. These changes, for better or worse, should be charted and reported to your supervisor.

Take some time to study those drugs most often used with LBD patients so that you'll be ahead of the game when you see them being used. Then, take a few moments to check out any new drugs so you can know what to expect from them.

Always remember, drugs shouldn't be considered the first line answer to behavioral issues. Even though you may not be responsible for deciding what drugs a patient takes, you still have the power to limit their need.

- Patients react automatically to the actions and attitudes of others.
- Your interaction with the patients can trigger negative or positive reactions.
- Negative reactions are likely to lead to the need for behavior management drugs.
- Positive reactions are more likely to lead to a happier, calmer more compliant patient.

Take classes and practice using non-drug methods. Many require nothing but acceptance, empathy and communication based on a basic understanding of how the dementia-damaged brain works.

End of Life Care

LBD is a progressively degenerative disease. Every LBD family eventually faces end of life issues and they need to know about palliative and hospice care. All professionals who work with dementia patients will likely work with these in some way, often regularly. Knowing about them, their functions and their limitations is a must if you want to provide the best care and support for your patients and their families.

29. Palliative Care

proactive dementia care: Care that focuses on helping a patient use their remaining skills to maintain independence and improve quality of life.

palliative dementia care: Care that focuses on comfort, peace and the relief of pain and suffering rather than maintaining skills or extending life.

***

A Change Of Focus

Nearing the end of life, a patient's needs change. Up to this time, they have needed a care partner and care staff who were cheerleaders, activity directors and more to keep them doing anything they could to extend their functionality. Dementia patients' care partners and families are encouraged to be aggressively proactive, pushing their loved ones to exercise, socialize, to eat right, sleep better at night and so on.

However, no matter how good the care, LBD is degenerative. Eventually the focus must change from proactive to palliative care; from doing everything to maintain a patient's skills to a gentler, more passive form of care.

Palliative care is compassionate care that focuses on peace and comfort rather than maintaining skills, on relieving stress and pain rather than maintaining health.

Hospice services often provide a service called "palliative care" for a minimal cost. Care partners will often choose this when they don't wish to accept the limitations required for hospice or when their loved ones don't yet qualify. It provides much the same care as hospice but a terminal diagnosis is not required and it is not covered by Medicare. However, Medicare may and often does pay for some specific palliative treatments such as pain drugs for a covered illness.

Care Partner Issues

The transition from a proactive to a palliative frame of mind can be difficult for care partners, especially if their focus has been intensely active. Accepting a more passive, relaxed mode of care can feel like giving up, accepting failure. Or they may be having difficulty accepting that the patient is actually in the stage of their life where hospice-provided palliative care is what they need most of all.

I've worked hard to help Peter stay as functional as he could be. But now the nurse tells me it is time for hospice. No! I don't want it to be that time. I don't want him to go yet. Yes, I know he is fading but he still has periods of awareness. Times when he holds my hand and looks at me with love. I'm not ready to give up yet. - Jenny Ellis

Jenny is voicing a common care partner misperception. The acceptance that a loved one has moved to a new stage and needs a different kind of care is not giving up. It is being willing to respond to the needs of their loved one rather than their own need for more time. Where once the care partner's encouragement to try, move and even to eat was the push the patient needed to overcome inertia, now it only adds stress.

Being proactive also helps the care partner maintain a feeling of control in a mostly uncontrollable situation. As such, it is hard to accept that all this activity and encouragement is no longer functional. Help them by giving the care partners and families new tasks. Explain that the job has changed again but remains equally important. Explain that now their job is one of finding and utilizing ways to decrease stress and increase comfort and companionship as their loved one travels this last stage of their journey.

It isn't only the family that must change focus. Treatment goals must change too. This is especially a concern with LBD, which causes so many physical problems in addition to the dementia. There comes a time when treatment for something even as life-threatening as kidney failure will make little difference—except to decrease the quality of one's final days. These treatments are usually stressful, which increases LBD symptoms and decreases quality of life without adding much if anything in the way of time. In fact, a patient subjected to stressful life-changing treatments will often die sooner than one who was not treated.

If they do live longer, their quality of life is likely going to be worse than it was before.

A common example of misguided care is the use of feeding tubes with an end-of-life dementia patient. Dementia is a debilitating disease. As the brain dies, so does the body—and its need for nourishment. The tube itself is uncomfortable, an unnecessary torture. Even worse, food that goes into a no longer functioning digestive system is likely to end in painful constipation.

30. Hospice

hospice care: Compassionate palliative care that includes the patient's physical, emotional and spiritual needs. This requires a doctor's statement that the end of life is near.

Medicare: A national health insurance that varies with each state but always includes hospice.

***

Hospice is a Medicare covered service that provides palliative treatment to qualified patients.[61] It is compassionate end-of-life medical, emotional and spiritual support provided by health professionals and volunteers. Its goal is to control pain and other symptoms so a person can remain as alert and comfortable as possible. Hospice programs also provide services to support a patient's family.

Eligibility

A patient is eligible for hospice covered by Medicare when:

- the person has Medicare Part A.
- their physician and a hospice medical director certifies a life expectancy of no longer than six months if the disease runs its normal course.
- the patient and their family elect to receive hospice care.

Financial coverage. Patients can receive hospice care without being on Medicare but they, or their insurance, will be responsible for payment of service.

Medicare certification. The six-months is an estimate not a requirement! Patients must be re-certified for benefits at various intervals:

- initially: Two 90-day periods
- followed by: Unlimited number of 60-day periods.

If found unqualified (too healthy!) to receive services, the patient will be removed from service but can go back on as soon as they meet the requirements again. It is not unusual for a person to go on and off several times.

Dementia specific qualifications. The National Hospice and Palliative Care Organization has published guidelines[62] to help identify a person with dementia who is within six months from the end of a normal course. With no other complications a person with dementia cannot:

- ambulate without assistance
- dress without assistance
- bathe properly
- control bowel and bladder
- speak more than half dozen or fewer intelligible and different words.

Usually, long before a LBD patient qualifies with the above criteria, they will have other complications, such as recurrent UTIs, aspiration pneumonia or other related problems that support a life expectancy of six months or less.

Location

Hospice care can take place in the patient's home, a hospice center or an adult care facility. It is less likely to take place in a hospital due to conflicts with the hospice non-life-extending policies. However, under some circumstances, it might.

Finding A Service

There are many in every community. The problem is less one of finding a hospice service than of finding the right one. For example, in the metropolitan Phoenix area, there are over 200 hospice groups. Some accept dementia patients and some don't. It is the same in most large communities. A list of hospice providers, their requirements and their services makes a good addition to your LBD library.

Cost

For any patient who is eligible for Medicare, hospice is free. It is included in all Medicare based insurance plans and is governed by Medicare regulations. If a patient does not qualify for Medicare, they may have insurance coverage. With no insurance, other arrangements can be made depending on the hospice group the family chooses.

However, even if the patient qualifies for free hospice care, not everything is free. The family may need to pay:

- $5 per prescription drug or other products for pain relief and symptom control.
- 5% of the Medicare-approved amount for inpatient respite care.
- all of residential facility fees. Medicare only pays for hospice services, not room and board.

Services

A hospice service staff includes:

- *health aides*, who help with bathing and other activities of daily living.
- *nurses,* who do house calls and make regular checks on the patient's condition.
- *volunteers,* who visit regularly and can stay with the patient while the care partner takes some "me time."
- *counselors and chaplains*, who offer emotional and spiritual support.
- *physicians*

Non-Patient Services

A hospice service isn't just for the patient. It is there to support the care partner as well. As noted earlier, anything that supports the care partner and makes their job easier--and their attitude more relaxed and happy-- supports the patient.

My sister Patricia is a typical 'old maid' with strong opinions that are often different from mine. It's not been easy living with her and I get so frustrated sometimes. That doesn't help my arthritis and I wasn't getting enough exercise either. When I shared my concerns with the hospice counselor, she started walking with me once a week while we talked about my issues. She listens to me vent so I can go back and care for my sister with more patience. She's been a true blessing! - Ellen

Hospice chaplains provide grief counseling, individually and in groups, before and after the patient has passed on. They understand that a dementia care partner goes through a lot of their grief long before their loved one is actually gone.

Special LBD Issues

Hospice staff will likely be trained to work with dementia patients but may know little about the special issues associated with LBD. While various kinds of dementia become more similar as the end nears, a couple of LBD specific issues remain.

Drug sensitivity. A LBD patient is apt to be sensitive to the drugs normally used by the hospice service for agitation and perhaps even for pain. For example, Haldol is an inexpensive antipsychotic and is often used by hospice services instead of more expensive ones such as Seroquel. LBD patients also can be sensitive to strong pain medication, especially in normal doses.

Showtime. This short period of temporary improvement can mask actual conditions at times when these conditions most need to be seen, such as when the hospice evaluator is there to affirm that the patient still qualifies for service.

Preparing For Hospice

Many people believe hospice service is for the last weeks or days of dying. Not so. Hospice is for the living, for making a person's last months as comfortable as possible. It should start as soon as the patient is eligible.

In fact, research for the right hospice service and discussions with the doctor about hospice should start well before the patient is eligible. This is not giving up or being negative. It is planning ahead. When the time comes, the family will likely be in crisis mode and this is not a time to be making plans. With a plan already in place, it just needs to be implemented.

Some doctors resist using hospice. They may see it as unnecessary bad news for their patients and family members. Or they may even see it as a failure on their part to keep their patient alive. These doctors are doing their patients a disservice by discouraging families from availing themselves of a multitude of help at a time when it is greatly needed. A care partner who lets the doctor know they are open to the idea of hospice allows the doctor to be open too.

Often a patient or family member will resist the idea of hospice because they don't want to face end of life issues.

My grandmother had mild LBD along with a serious heart problem. When her doctor suggested hospice, she wanted to change doctors. Grandma told us "The doctor told me I had to die in six months if I accepted hospice care. Well, I'm not ready to die!" Mom checked with the staff and a nurse went in and talked to Grandma. She told her that the doctor's words were an estimate, not a requirement. Grandma agreed to accept and she actually lived on hospice for a whole 18 months. We were so grateful for the whole program. Grandma liked all the extra attention and the family liked the caring attitude of the workers. - Lee, an online group member

As the nurse did with Lee's grandmother and her family, encourage the family to view hospice positively, as an added physical and emotional support during a time when both are sorely needed. The lowered levels of stress often result in better health for the patient, thus hospice can actually be considered proactive! You can also assure them that hospice is voluntary. A family can choose to take a loved one off hospice at any time. This change of view and sense of control may help move them from their ingrained proactive stance to one of relaxed compassion.

A care partner should ask questions like the following when researching which hospice service to use:

- What services do you provide?
- Where do you provide services?
- Who provides them? What are the provider's qualifications? For example are the nurses RNs or LPNs? Is the doctor an MD or do you use Nurse Practitioners or a Physician's Assistants?
- Do you use volunteers? What are they allowed to do? How are they vetted? What kind of training do they receive?
- How familiar are you with the LBD patient's sensitivity to certain medications, including many strong pain medications and especially first generation antipsychotics (Haldol)?

- Which of my loved one's medications are considered palliative and which, if any, are not? What will happen about those that are not?
- What do you know about LBD and its fluctuations, including Showtime?
- How much dementia training does the staff receive?
- How much of the training is specific to LBD? For example, do you teach about LBD's fluctuations, including Showtime? Do you teach about LBD's drug sensitivities, including that to traditional psychotics such as Haldol?

This pre-work is especially important with LBD. Fluctuations are normal symptoms but an unexpected infection, injury or illness can cause a sharp downturn from which the patient never recovers. This may send them into the last phase of their illness, where hospice needs to be considered well before the family may have thought it would be needed.

Making The Decision To Go On Hospice

Hospice care is palliative, not curative. Patient and family must agree to use only palliative medications, those that provide the patient with pain relief and comfort. Many of a dementia patient's medications do just this. However, others may not be considered palliative and may have to be dropped to meet the criteria. The description of what is considered palliative and what is not can vary with the service.

This can be a sticking point with some care partners for several reasons.

- It difficult for them to consider dropping a drug they know has been life-extending for their loved one. They may not have transitioned from a proactive mode of care to a supportive, comforting mode of care. It is part of the care staff's job to help care partners and families take this painful step and see that it is what their loved one needs at this time of their life.
- The hospice service demands that certain long-helpful drugs be ended as unnecessary. For example, dementia drugs, once very helpful, tend to lose ineffectiveness eventually and so their removal is likely appropriate. Patients don't need unnecessary drugs and will do better without these drugs in their system.

Accepting this is part of the move from proactive care to comforting care.

- The hospice service demands the removal of life-extending drugs that the family sees as also being otherwise helpful. For example, those for treatment of heart-related problems may also decrease pain or anxiety while doing their primary job. Other more hospice acceptable drugs can often be substituted to provide this palliative support.

- The hospice service requires that a drug such as Seroquel be replaced by a less expensive but more LBD-sensitive antipsychotic such as Haldol. This is something a care partner needs to know prior to using hospice. These drugs are seldom compatible with LBD.

Before a family chooses a hospice service, they need to interview the ones in their area to find the one that best fits their needs. It isn't unusual to have hundreds of hospice service organizations in each metropolitan area. While Medicare's requirements are firm, each service interprets them differently, just as each insurance company does.

Care partners who cannot find a hospice service that meets their needs can often opt to use palliative care instead and pay for the extra costs not covered by Medicare.

Going Off--And Back On--Hospice

Patients get such good care on hospice that they often do improve so much that they no longer qualify for hospice service. This isn't a major crisis however. As soon as their health degenerates again, they can go back on the service.

A family may choose to remove their loved one from hospice at any time as well. For example, they may want to pursue a treatment that the hospice service can't support. This might happen when a patient has a heart attack. Most hospice services have a respite center where patients who need more acute care can stay instead of going to a hospital. If the family prefers hospital care, this is considered life-extending treatment and the patient would have to go off hospice.

Once the patient again qualifies for hospice, they can return. In some cases this would mean when they begin to degenerate again. In others, it might mean when the patient and family are again willing to accept hospice limitations. In the case of hospitalization, the patient would likely qualify for hospice once hospitalization was no longer necessary. There is no penalty for going off hospice and no limit to the number of times a patient can go on or off.

Grieving

Grieving for a patient with dementia usually starts long before death. As the disease takes more and more of a loved one, care partners and families experience anticipatory grief. They grieve for the person that was and for what is coming. Often, by the time the patient dies, the family is feeling more relief than grief, relief that the ordeal is over for both the patient and themselves. A care partner often refers to this as their loved one is free of Lewy's grip or that they won their battle against Lewy.

Wherever the family is in their grief, it is the care staff's job to support them and provide them with referrals for grief counseling. If you deal with dying patients, you probably need counseling too. You may not have the long-term attachment with them that the family does but they have become persons to you and you likely have some feelings about them as they pass.

Care partners may express guilt about feelings of relief. Help them to see that this is a normal part of the process and nothing to feel guilty about. Help them to see that it is about the ending of a job well done.

Hospice services always offer grief counseling, individually and in groups. Encourage the care partner and grieving family members to attend.

Appendix

History

It isn't really important that you know the history of how LBD was discovered and became accepted as a "disease." It probably isn't going to change how you deal with it or treat it. However, for those of you who are interested in that sort of thing...as the authors were...here it is:

LBD is the second most common degenerative dementia, after Alzheimer's. There are at least 1.5 million cases of diagnosed LBD in this country.[63] It is considered to be grossly under-diagnosed and/or misdiagnosed as other diseases, thus the true number is likely much higher. So then, if so many people have LBD, then one might think that it would be fairly well known. Not so. Both forms of LBD have had a rocky road to acceptance as "real" dementias for which a physician can bill insurances and drug companies can advertise dementia medications.

The Road To Acceptance
Dementia With Lewy Bodies (DLB)

In 1912, Dr. Fredrick Lewy, a colleague of Dr. Alzheimer in Germany, was looking at tissues from brain autopsies, searching for the cause of Parkinson's disease. He reported seeing abnormal protein structures in the substantia nigra.[64] Not much happened however, until the 1970's when researchers in Japan, led by Dr. Kenji Kosaka, discovered the same abnormal proteins in the cerebral cortex and named them Lewy bodies after Dr. Lewy.[65] In 1984, Dr. Kosaka published a paper connecting Lewy bodies in the cerebral cortex with dementia symptoms a patient demonstrated prior to death. This article was the first description of "dementia with Lewy bodies."[66]

Although scientists and neurologists developed a gradual awareness of this "new" type of dementia, it was seldom diagnosed because it had no formal diagnostic criteria. Finally, in 1994, dementia specialists met at the First International Workshop on DLB and devised a set of formal DLB clinical diagnostic criteria, published that same year.[67]

One might also think that finally, with an accepted set of diagnostic criteria, DLB would become better known. However, getting a "new" disease recognized is a long and cumbersome process and developing the diagnostic criteria is only the first step. For DLB, that first step took over a decade from Dr. Kosaka's description in 1984 to an agreement among recognized specialists in 1994.

Once a disease has formal recognition, a report must be written and submitted to an appropriate journal. Since such a report is usually a cooperative effort between specialists living in widely separated geographic locations, with greatly varied ideas and often, equally large egos, it can be months in the making. Once submitted, it may be a year before a journal can publish the article. For DLB, this part of the process was comparatively short: only a little more than a year from the meeting in 1994 to the published article in 1996.

The next step is to get a code for the disease listed in the International Classification of Diseases (ICD). This manual provides billing codes for insurance companies. No billing code; no payment. Until there is a code, many physicians diagnose a billable disease like Alzheimer's, even in the presence of symptoms that clearly meet the diagnostic criteria for a disease with no code. Depending on a variety of issues including when the next revision is planned, obtaining a code for a new disease can take several years. The ICD-version 9 (ICD-9) finally listed "331.82: dementia with Lewy bodies" in 2004, eight years after the diagnostic criteria for DLB was published.[68] In the ICD-10, it is listed as G31.83.

The third step is to get the disease listed in the Diagnostic and Statistical Manual of Mental Disorders (DSM). The Food and Drug Administration (FDA), which approves drugs for use with specific diseases, uses this code book rather than the ICD for brain related diseases. Until a dementia is listed in this book, no drugs can be approved for it. This list was last revised in 1994, two years before DLB had a formal diagnosis criteria. In 2013, a long-promised revision from DSM-IV to DSM-5 finally included a code for Dementia with Lewy bodies.[69] Prior to that, many physicians diagnosed clearly identifiable DLB as Alzheimer's to avoid "off-label"[e] issues with insurance companies. As of mid 2019, no drugs specifically for DLB are on the market but some are in clinical trial stages.

Parkinson's Disease With Dementia (PDD)

As a well-known symptom of Parkinson's disease, PDD has had both ICD-9 and DSM-IV codes for many years. However, PD is a movement disorder, treated by movement disorder specialists and the dementia component of the disease was seldom addressed specifically.

Until 2007, there were no drugs approved for use with the dementia symptoms of PD although it was becoming clear that like DLB, PDD responded even better than Alzheimer's to many dementia drugs. Then, in 2006, a group of dementia and movement specialists met and agreed that PDD and DLB were so similar that their cognitive aspects could be treated identically.[70] Soon afterward, in 2007, movement specialists published diagnostic criteria for PDD which is very similar to that for DLB.[71]

With PDD identified as a specific dementia and a DSM-IV code already in place, drug companies could design drugs for this disease. By the end of 2007, two companies were advertising dementia drugs for PDD patients. This portion of the Lewy body dementias can now be treated specifically without resorting to using off-label drugs or misdiagnosing to avoid the off-label quandary.[e]

In June 2017 the international Dementia with Lewy Bodies (DLB) Consortium published updated diagnostic criteria for dementia with Lewy bodies.[72]

The criteria is now divided between clinical features (subjective physical symptoms) and biomarkers (objective tests). These are divided again according to their strength for a diagnosis. Core clinical features and indicative biomarkers are given more weight. Supportive features and supportive biomarkers are considered just that: supportive but not strong enough to be used alone for a diagnosis.

---

[e] **Off-label drugs**: Those not approved by the Food and Drug administration (FDA) for the specific disease for which they are prescribed. Insurances may not pay for off-label drugs.

Other changes involve:

- Giving more weight to RBD and to the MIBG biomarker.
- The addition of hypersomnia (excessive sleeping) and hyposmia (poor sense of smell) as new supportive clinical features.

This new diagnosis follows in the footsteps of older ones in recognizing that DLB is a multi-system, multi-symptom disorder and that no two patients will express it in the same way.

Formal 2017 DLB Diagnostic Criteria

This is the revised criteria for the clinical diagnosis of probable and possible DLB as published by the DLB Consortium. (The criteria in Chapter 5 is a simplified version.)

Clinical Features

Essential Feature: Required For A DLB Diagnosis.

Dementia, defined as a progressive cognitive decline of sufficient magnitude to interfere with normal social or occupational functions, or with usual daily activities.

- Prominent or persistent memory impairment may not necessarily occur in the early stages but is usually evident with progression.
- Deficits on tests of attention, executive function and visuo-perceptual ability may be especially prominent and occur early.

Core Clinical Features

(NOTE: The first 3 typically occur early and may persist throughout the course of the disease.)

Fluctuating cognition with pronounced variations in attention and alertness

Recurrent visual hallucinations that are typically well formed and detailed

REM sleep behavior disorder (RBD) which may precede cognitive decline

One or more spontaneous cardinal feature of parkinsonism – these are bradykinesia (defined as slowness of movement and decrement in amplitude or speed), rest tremor, or rigidity.

Supportive Clinical Features

Severe sensitivity to antipsychotic agents; postural instability; repeated falls; syncope or other transient episodes of unresponsiveness; severe autonomic dysfunction e.g. constipation, orthostatic hypotension, urinary incontinence; hypersomnia; hyposmia; hallucinations in other modalities; systematized delusions; apathy, anxiety and depression.

Biomarkers

Indicative Biomarkers

A. Reduced dopamine transporter (DaT) uptake in basal ganglia demonstrated by SPECT or PET
B. Abnormal (low uptake) 123iodine- MIBG myocardial scintigraphy
C. Polysomnographic confirmation of REM sleep without atonia

Supportive Biomarkers

A. Relative preservation of medial temporal lobe structures on CT/MRI scan
B. Generalized low uptake on SPECT/PET perfusion/metabolism scan with reduced occipital activity +/- the cingulate island sign on FDG-PET imaging
C. Prominent posterior slow wave activity on EEG with periodic fluctuations in the pre-alpha/theta range

Probable Or Possible DLB Diagnostic Formula

Probable DLB:

A. two or more core clinical features of DLB are present, with or without the presence of indicative biomarkers **or**
B. only one core clinical feature is present, but with one or more indicative biomarkers.

Probable DLB should not be diagnosed on the basis of biomarkers alone.

Possible DLB:

A. only one core clinical feature of DLB is present, with no indicative biomarker evidence, **or**
B. one or more indicative biomarkers is present but there are no core clinical features

DLB Is Less Likely:

in the presence of any other physical illness or brain disorder including cerebrovascular disease, sufficient to account in part or in total for the clinical picture, although these do not exclude a DLB diagnosis and may serve to indicate mixed or multiple pathologies contributing to the clinical presentation, or

if parkinsonian features are the only core clinical feature and appear for the first time at a stage of severe dementia.

Biomarkers and Imaging Processes

Biomarkers

A biomarker is a substance in the body that can be used as an objective diagnostic tool that indicates the presence and severity of a condition or disease. Biomarkers can be measured, repeated and validated--or discounted. Most of us are familiar with blood, urine and saliva tests that use biomarkers to indicate a variety of conditions from pregnancy to strep throat to HIV and much more. A biomarker can be a cell or tissue in the body already, such as the blood sugar of a diabetic but a brain-related (neurological) biomarker is usually a tiny amount of an inserted, target-specific substance, called a radio-active tracer. It goes deep into the body tissues to its targeted area and then exits the body within 48 hours.

Imaging devices follow the tracer's progress and measure its interaction with targeted cells to provide information about diseases like DLB that until recently, could only be obtained via an autopsy after the person died. Biomarkers measure Lewy body activity and the results of this activity rather than the actual Lewy bodies themselves. Thus, their information alone is not considered conclusive. They do add to the likelihood of an accurate diagnosis, even for the less Lewy-savvy doctor.

The hope of the future. Neurological biomarkers can reach inside cells to find early, minute signs of a disease before it grows too big to eliminate, that is, well before there are symptoms. Many people are now living healthy lives after being treated for a cancer that was found while it was still small enough to treat successfully. That is still not possible with neurological diseases like DLB. However, now that biomarkers can identify small groups of Lewy bodies, researchers can look for ways to stop them from expanding.

Brain Imaging

Autopsy. An autopsy is the only accepted conclusive test for a Lewy body disease. Because one must use an electron microscope to see Lewy bodies, it can only be done during brain autopsies. Although this

193

has greatly improved LBD research and has added to our basic knowledge about the disorder, it is of no help to the live patient seeking a diagnosis.

Live brain scans.[73] While effective, these scanners and the tracers the tests require are expensive to acquire and maintain and costly to use. In addition, they are not readily available in the US. They can usually be found in research and teaching centers but are less likely anywhere else. This and the fact that they are still not accepted as 100% conclusive makes some physicians regard them as optional or even unnecessary for a diagnosis. And they can be. If the clinical features are already there, the diagnosis is probably not going to change. If there is only one clinical feature, then the imaging might make a difference.

However, if the need for a diagnosis is mainly to assure that a person with a Lewy body disease is not given drugs that might trigger their drug sensitivities, then even a "possible" DLB diagnosis is enough. Any more could be considered a waste of time and money--and an unnecessary hardship on the patient and their family.

These two brain imaging processes both use radio-active tracers:

- Positron Emission Tomography (PET scan). A 3-D imaging process that uses a radio-active tracer to measure brain cell functioning.
- Single-Photon Emission Computed Tomography (SPECT scan). A 3-D imaging process that uses a radio-active tracer to measure electrical activity in the brain.

This 2-D heart imaging process also uses radio-active tracers:

- Scintigraphy (Gamma): A gamma camera tracks and measures a tracer's gamma rays to provide 2-D information about internal body organs. Gamma rays are electromagnetic radiation similar to x-rays except that, with a shorter wavelength and higher energy, they are more penetrating.

These more complex tests are often combined with these more common imaging processes to produce even better 3-D images of how a cell is functioning:

- Computerized tomography (CT scan). Combines a series of X-ray images taken from different angles around your body and uses computer processing to create cross-sectional images (slices) of the brain or other organs.
- Magnetic resonance imaging (MRI scan). Uses a large magnet and radio waves to look inside the brain, heart or other organs.

This next process measures electrical activity in the brain:

- Electroencephalography (EEG). Uses electrodes to measure brain waves and activity in various parts of the brain.

Imaging Tests Used In The 2017 Criteria

Each test uses one or more of the above processes. If a tracer is used, the test is usually named for that tracer.[74]

DaT scan: Uses the ^{123}I-FP-CIT tracer to detect dopamine (DA) activity in brain cells, which varies determining on which dementia is present, Alzheimer's or LBD. DaT scans were only available in Europe but with their inclusion in the 2017 DLB criteria, they have become available in some U.S. research and teaching centers. (Indicative Biomarker A)

MIBG scan:[75] A gamma scan that uses the ^{123}I-meta-iodobenzylguanidine (MIBG) tracer to measure evidence of damage to nerves in the heart that control several autonomic functions like heart beat and blood pressure. MIBG scans are available in most cities, usually at a lower cost than scans requiring PET or SPECT equipment. (Indicative Biomarker B)

FDG-PET scan:[76] Uses the [18]fluorine-fluorodeoxyglucose (FDG) tracer to measure the brain's ability to metabolize sugar. LBD patients who hallucinate tend to have decreased brain metabolism in the occipital (visual) lobe of the brain, compared to that of a person with Alzheimer's. FDG PET is available as a diagnostic tool in the US and is covered under Medicare under certain conditions. (Supportive Biomarker B)

Structural imaging: CT or MRI scans are used without tracers to scan the brain for structural damage or lack thereof. Structural imaging is comparatively inexpensive and available in most cities. (Supportive Biomarker A)

Coherence analysis: EEG waves are measured and compared by computer to look for physical evidence of periodic fluctuations in brain functionality (coherence). (Supportive Biomarker C)

Resources

Alternative Therapy Information

Acupressure for Beginners. (exploreim.ucla.edu/self-care /acupressure-and-common-acupressure-points/) UCLA's Center for East-West Medicine blog on Integrative Medicine explains how acupressure works and offers some basic directions for use. Is not specific to dementia.

Alternative Therapies. (lbdtools.com/alternative-therapies.php) Alternative therapy consultant Regina Huck's large section on a variety of alternative options for use with people living with dementia.

An Introductory Guide to 1000's of Uses for Essential Oils. (sustainablebabysteps.com/uses-for-essential-oils.html) Provides a good basic reference, listing oils alphabetically with their functions and identifying the qualities of a "good oil" without naming a brand.

Complementary and Alternative Treatments for Dementia. (verywellhealth.com/complementary-and-alternative-therapies-for-dementia-98671) An overview by Esther Heerem of non-drug options that can be used with or without drugs for people living with dementia.

Essential Oils. (wholenewmom.com/health-concerns/natural-remedies/the-great-essential-oils-showdown-in-search-of-the-best-essential-oils/) Whole New Mom blogger Adrienne's well researched six-part blog on essential oils, how to choose them, which company she prefers and why.

The Role of Massage Therapy in Dementia Care. (massagetoday.com/mpacms/mt/article.php?id=15057) Women in Bodywork blogger Ann Catlin's overview of how to use massage to help a person living with dementia feel less pain, anxiety,etc.

Blogs And Websites

LBDtools.com: The Whitworth's website, filled with LBD info and care suggestions.

Lewy Body Roller Coaster: (lewybodydementia.blogspot.com) The Whitworth's weekly blog about all aspects of Lewy body care partnering. Blogs accessible from 2011 to the present.

Lewybodydementia.ca: A Canadian website hosted by Timothy Hudson that offers a wide variety of valuable information.

Teepa Snow: Positive Approach to Brain Change. (teepasnow.com) A great source of information and training for care partners and staff. We can personally recommend Teepa Snow's work.

Brain Donation Sites

Brain Support Network. (brainsupportnetwork.org) Contact this group first. They provide complete, detailed brain donation arrangements and support the entire way, tailored to the specific person, their location and their diagnosis. robin.riddle@brainsupportnetwork.org, 650.814.0848

Banner Sun Health Research Institute. (bannerhealth.com/ways-to-give/organ-donation) Sun City, AZ. 833.252.5535.

Boston University School of Medicine, (bu.edu/alzresearch/education-resources/ethnicity/donation/) Alzheimer's Disease Center. Boston, MA. 888.458.2823.

Northwestern University, Chicago, IL *(brain.northwestern.edu/pdfs/controlautopsy.pdf)* 312.926.1851.

University of California. (memory.ucsf.edu/research-trials/brain-donation) Memory and Aging Center. San Francisco, CA. 415.476.1681.

Caregiver Information

Aging and Disability in America. *(acl.gov/aging-and-disability-in-america)* Directory to government programs at bottom of page.

Assist Guide Information Center. *(agis.com)* Caregiver information, support, checklists and databases, information.

Caregiver Action Network. (caregiveraction.org) Their Caregiver Toolkit contains many guides such as Managing Medication or Financial Planning. Help line: 855-227-3640.

Disability.gov. *(dol.gov/odep/topics/disability.htm)* Guide to many comprehensive disability-related government resources.

Family Caregiver Alliance. (*caregiver.org*) Excellent source of caregiver information. Search by state for multiple local resources. 800.445.8106.

National Association of Area Agencies on Aging. (*n4a.org*) A directory to a variety of services to seniors with local offices in most areas. 202.872.8888, email: info@n4a.org.

SeniorLiving.org. Includes helpful guides on money, housing and health care

USA.gov for Seniors. (*usa.gov/features/usagovs-guide-for-seniors*) Directory to federal and state agencies and sites that provide a wide variety of services for seniors. 844.USA.GOV1.

Drug Information

AARP Health Tools. (*healthtools.aarp.org/drug-directory*) Search for drugs, check interactions, compare drugs and identify pills. AARP Health Tools also has a symptom checker.

MedlinePlus: (*nlm.nih.gov/medlineplus/druginformation.html*) Search for drugs, herbs and supplements, by generic or brand name.

WebMD: Search for drugs, vitamins and supplements. identify pills and check drug interactions.

Drugs.com. Pill checker with photos. Drug interaction checker that lists all interactions for a single drug with severity, checks for interactions between an individualized list of drugs and accumulates information from successive searches.

LBDA Medical Alert Wallet Card. (*lbda.org/content/lbd-medical-alert-wallet-card*) Carry this card with you everywhere.

Publications for Professionals. (*lbda.org/physicians*) A list of articles and checklists designed especially for professionals. Good articles to copy and share with other professionals.

Treating Psychosis in LBD. (*lbda.org/go/ER*) Download this and keep it handy for emergencies.

Anticholinergic Drug Lists

Senior List. (*theseniorlist.com/medication/anticholinergic-drugs/*) List of Anticholinergic Drugs and Why Some of Them are Dangerous for Seniors. Updated 1/12/2019.

Updated American Geriatrics Society Beers Criteria® for Potentially Inappropriate Medication Use in Older Adults. (Stored in: *qioprogram.org › sites › default › files › 2019BeersCriteria_JAGS*) Revised from the 2015 list, this is considered the gold standard of these lists.

Financial Assistance Programs

Benefits.gov. Free confidential tool to help individuals find government benefits they may be eligible to receive.

Hilarity for Charity. (*hilarityforcharity.org*) Nonprofit that raises money for grants for dementia caregiver assistance. Online email application form for grant to help with home care.

Medicare.gov. The Official U.S. government site for people with Medicare.

Rebuilding Together. (*rebuildingtogether.org*) National nonprofit for low/no cost home modifications. 120 local offices. 800-473-4229

Social Security Administration. (*ssa.gov*). Information and resources including databases and publications. 800.772.1213: live M-F, 7AM to 7PM EST. Recorded information and services are available 24/7.

Veterans Administration. (*va.gov*) Information on VA benefits and services such as Aid & Attendance. 800.827.1000.

Home Safety

Assist Guide Information Services (AGIS) (*agis.com/eldercare-basics/Staying-at-Home/Improving-your-home/*). Includes several safety checklists. 866.511.9186.

National Institute on Aging. (NIA) (*nia.nih.gov/health/home-safety-checklist-alzheimers-disease*) Thorough home safety checklist.

LBD Specific Treatment

Alzheimer's Disease Research Centers (ADRC): (*nia.nih.gov/health/alzheimers-disease-research-centers*) Medical centers identified by the NIH as centers specializing in Alzheimer's *and other dementias.* 602-839-6900

Research Centers of Excellence (RCOE): (*lbda.org/rcoe*) Medical centers certified by the LBDA to treat LBD.

Legal Help

AARP. Advance Directive Forms. (*aarp.org/caregiving/financial-legal/free-printable-advance-directives/*) Free download by state.

The National Academy of Elder Law Attorneys, Inc. (NAELA). (*naela.org/findlawyer*). Find eldercare lawyers in your city, state or zip code.

U.S. Living Will Registry. (*uslwr.com/formslist.shtm*) Advance directive forms by state. Offers a $5 registry program helpful if you travel a lot.

Long-Term Care And Placement

A Place for Mom. (*aplaceformom.com*) Senior care by state. Offers free personalized recommendations.

Carelike Care Seeker: (*careseeker.carelike.com*) Directory of various care options by city and state.

Veterans Geriatrics and Extended Care. (*va.gov/GERIATRICS*) Information about VA supported home, community based and residential long term care options.

LongTermCare.gov: The official US Government site for long term care information.

Nursing Home Comparison. (*medicare.gov/NHCompare/search.html*) Detailed information about the past performance of every Medicare and Medicaid certified nursing home in the country.

Support Organizations

Lewy Body Dementia

Lewy Body Dementia Association (*lbda.org*) An excellent source of LBD Caregiver information and support. Many local support groups. Caregiver help line: 800.539.9767. Office: 404.935.6444.

Lewy Body Resource Center. (*lewybodyresourcecenter.org/*) A New York based group offering LBD resources and information nationwide.

Lewy Body Society (*lewybody.org/*) UK organization with good general information.

Dementia Australia. (*dementia.org.au/resources/lewy-body-resources*) Australian site with good information and resources.

LBD Support Groups

Most are closed groups. You must apply and be accepted as a member.

Caring Spouses Group (*groups.io/g/LBDCaringSpouses*) Limited to spouses of LBD patients. Email link for joining group: LBDCaringSpouses+subscribe@groups.io

Lewy Body Carers (*facebook.com/groups/lyndseywilliams*) For anyone affected by LBD--individuals, family, friends.

Lewy Body Dementia Care Partner Support Group. (*facebook.com/groups/LBDACarePartnerSupportGroup*) For care partners of those living with LBD.

Lewy Body Dementia Caregivers Support Group. (*facebook.com/groups/LewyBodyDementiaCaregiversSupportGroup*) For caregivers of those living with LBD.

Lewy Body Support Group. For care partners and patients. (*facebook.com/groups/LewyBodySupportGroup*)

Alzheimer's Disease

Alzheimer's Association. (*alz.org*) Nationwide Local Chapters and Caregiver Support Groups. Helpline: 800.272.3900.

Alzheimer's Foundation of America. (*alzfdn.org*) Social Worker Helpline: 866.232.8484. (Also available via Skype, live chat or email.)

Alzheimer's and Related Dementias Education and Referral (ADEAR) (*nia.nih.gov/health/about-adear-center*) A current, comprehensive, unbiased source of information about Alzheimer's disease and related dementias.

Early-Onset Dementia

Living Together with Lewy Facebook Support Group. (*facebook.com/groups/LBDALivingTogetherwithLewy/*) For those living with LBD and their care partners.

Living with Lewy Facebook Support Group.
(*facebook.com/groups/LBDALivingwithLewy/*) For those living with LBD with or without a diagnosis.

Young Onset Dementia Support Page.
(*facebook.com/YoungOnsetDementiaSupportPage/*) A public site for those experiencing the impact of dementia before age 65.

Frontotemporal Disorders

The Association for Frontotemporal Degeneration. (*theaftd.org*) Provides accurate information, compassion and hope when lives are touched by any type of FTD. Email: info@theaftd.org. Helpline: 866.507.7222.

Parkinson's Disease

Besides the organizations listed here, there are multiple regional PD organizations. Ask your local Area Agency on Aging representative.

American Parkinson Disease Association. (*apdaparkinson.org*) Information and referral centers in many states. Lists PD health centers by state. Email: apda@apdaparkinson.org. 718.981.8001 or 800.223.2732

Michael J. Fox Foundation for Parkinson's Research.
(*michaeljfox.org*) Funding research is primary function. 212.509.0995

Parkinson's Foundation. (*parkinson.org*) Research, education and outreach.. Email: contact@parkinson.org. Helpline: 800-4PD-INFO (473-4636)

The Parkinson's Institute and Clinical Center. (thepi.org) Treatment and research. Email: info@thepi.org. (650) 770-0201.

Glossary of Terms

-A-

acceptance: Accepting another person's *reality* without necessarily believing it.

acetylcholine (ACh): A chemical compound in neurons that acts as a neurotransmitter and carries information between two nerve cells. A key neurotransmitter in the brain cortex, facilitating cognition.

acetylcholinesterase: The specific type of cholinesterase that breaks down acetylcholine. (See cholinesterase)

Active Dreams: A care partner's descriptive name for REM Sleep Behavior Disorder (RBD) borrowed to use in this book.

activities of daily living (ADLs): Personal care activities necessary for everyday living such as eating, bathing, grooming, dressing, mobility and toileting. A person's amount of dementia is sometimes measured by these limitations.

adult daycare: Place where adults living at home can go during the day for activities, socializing, education, physical therapy and health care, providing participants opportunities to interact with others while providing respite time for a care partner.

adverse drug reaction: Unexpected, unwanted or dangerous reaction to a drug, usually just the opposite of the usual effect. The onset of the adverse reaction may be sudden or develop over time. Also termed adverse effect or adverse event.

agitation: Excessive motor activity associated with a feeling of inner tension. Can be seen as verbal and physical aggression, active resistance to care, pacing, fidgeting, hand wringing, pulling of clothes and the inability to sit still.

agnosia: Inability to recognize and identify objects or persons despite having knowledge of the characteristics of those objects or persons. People with agnosia may retain their cognitive abilities in other areas.

aggression: Hostile or violent behavior towards another, often expressed in response to unintentionally triggering of residual negative feelings.

akathisia: Movement disorder characterized by a feeling of inner restlessness and a compelling need to be in constant motion such as fidgeting.

akinesia: Impaired body movement; without movement (or without much movement). Akinesia is a term used in neurology to denote the absence of movement.

alpha-synuclein: One in a family of structurally related proteins that are prominently expressed in the central nervous system.

Alzheimer's Disease: Progressive neurodegenerative disease of the brain.

Ambien (zolpidem tartrate): Sedative hypnotic drug used to treat patients with insomnia. It is associated with an increased risk for dementia in the elderly and not recommended for use with LBD. (See sedative hypnotic drugs)

ambulatory care: Medical care including diagnosis, observation, treatment and rehabilitation that is provided on an outpatient basis to persons who are able to ambulate or walk about.

ambulatory: Able to ambulate, to walk about. Not bed-ridden.

amino acids: Organic compounds that serve as building blocks for proteins.

amnesia: Forgetfulness for details of recent events, conversations and upcoming appointments.

amyloid precursor protein (APP): Gene when mutated that causes an abnormal form of the amyloid protein to be produced.

amyloid: Any of a number of complex proteins that can be deposited in tissues including organ specific areas such as the central nervous system, as in Alzheimer's, Parkinson's, Huntington's and Lewy body disease.

anticholinergic effect: A chemical effect that interferes with or lessens memory and thinking functions and may increase sleepiness and risks for imbalance or falling.

anxiety: Abnormal and overwhelming sense of apprehension and fear, often marked by sweating, tension and increased pulse, that affect everyday functioning.

apathy: Lack of motivation to initiate conversations or perform activities.

aphasia: Deterioration of the language function, resulting in an inability to comprehend speech. Sometimes considered a severe form of dysphasia.

apologizing: A great tool for deflecting anger.

Aricept (donepezil hydrochloride): A cholinesterase inhibitor to treat mild to moderate dementia.

assisted living facility: Long-term care facility with on-call nursing staff for individuals who are independent but need help with some activities of daily living.

ataxia: Wobbliness and unsteadiness due to the brain's failure to regulate the body's posture and regulate the strength and direction of limb movements.

atrophy: Decrease in size or wasting away of a body part or tissue.

attention deficit: the inability to ignore distractions and pay attention to a specific event, resulting in impulsive behavior and excessive activity.

attention: The ability to stay focused and to ignore distractions.

autonomic functions: Body functions that the brain controls via the autonomic nervous system without a person's conscious attention. Includes gland function, heart rate, digestion, respiratory rate, pupil size, urination and sexual arousal.

autonomic nervous system (ANS): The part of the nervous system that regulates the autonomic functions of the body. The ANS is divided into several systems including the inhibitory and excitatory systems. LBD can cause increased inhibitory effects and a decrease of excitatory effects, thus causing a slowing down of involuntary functions. (see inhibitory system and excitatory system)

-B-

Bad Times: Times when a patient is more confused, as compared to Good Times or Showtimes. (See fluctuating cognition.)

behaviors, dementia-related: Behaviors due to dementia or dementia symptoms such as delusions.

behaviors, non-disruptive: Those dementia-related behaviors that may distress the care partner but do not distress the patient.

black box warning: FDA required warning on all antipsychotic product packaging[77] that the use of antipsychotics in the elderly is linked to increased risk of serious illness and death.

body systems: Circulatory, immune, skeletal, urinary, muscular, hormonal, digestive, nervous and respiratory.

bradykinesia: Slowness of movement.

bradyphrasia: Slowness of thought.

brain stem: Stem-like part of the brain that is connected to the spinal cord. The brain stem manages messages going between the brain and the rest of the body, autonomic nervous system functions, consciousness and sleep cycles. The substantia nigra is located in this area.

bribe: Offering something pleasant to move the patient away from unwelcome activity. A very efficient distraction tool to use with someone experiencing dementia but not recommended for anyone who can learn to manipulate, such as children.

-C-

Capgras syndrome: A delusional misidentification where the patient believes that someone close to them (spouse, care partner) has been replaced by a similar-appearing imposter.

carbamazepine: See Tegretol.

carbidopa: Drug used together with Parkinson's drug, levodopa, to reduce its side-effects of nausea and vomiting. Has anticholinergic properties. (See Sinemet)

care partner: Individual who cares for others who have health problems or disabilities.

catheter: Hollow flexible tube, inserted into a body cavity, duct, or vessel to allow the passage of fluids or distend a passageway.

CBD oil: Cannabidiol (CBD) is an essential component of medical marijuana. It is believed to have many healing properties including pain relief and anxiety management without the hallucinogen properties of THC.

Celebrex (celecoxib): An anti-inflammatory drug thought to reduce dementia risk in persons with a family history of dementia.

celecoxib: See Celebrex.

Celexa (citalopram hydrobromide): SSRI antidepressant medication.

central nervous system (CNS): Part of the nervous system consisting of the brain and spinal cord.

cerebral cortex: A thin layer of the brain that covers the cerebrum with functions involved in the processes of thought, perception and memory, advanced motor function, social abilities, language and problem solving.

cerebral: Pertaining to the brain, the cerebrum or the intellect.

cerebrospinal fluid: Watery fluid, continuously produced and absorbed, which flows in the cavities within the brain and around the surface of the brain and spinal cord.

cerebrovascular disease: AKA stroke. Disease of the *cerebrum* and the blood vessels supplying it. Symptoms include dementia.

cerebrovascular: System of blood vessels and arteries that supply the brain.

cerebrum: The front part of the brain involved with thought, decision, emotion, character and voluntary actions.

change: A removal of the familiar and a threat to security.

chloral hydrate: A mild sedative hypnotic long used as a sleeping aid for insomnia. Has not been tested for safety with LBD.

cholinesterase: AKA acetylcholinesterase. An enzyme that breaks down the neurotransmitter, acetylcholine, so that it does not over-stimulate post-synaptic nerves, muscles and exocrine glands.

citalopram hydrobromide: See Celexa.

clinical trials: Trials to evaluate the effectiveness and safety of medications or medical devices by monitoring their effects on large groups of people over time.

clonazepam: See Klonopin.

cognition: The use of one's cognitive abilities.(See cognitive abilities.)

cognitive abilities: Memory, thinking, perceptual, attention and impulse control skills used for intellectual activity.

cognitive fluctuations: See fluctuating cognition.

comfort: A positive feeling of being relaxed, unworried and free from emotional or physical pain.

computerized axial tomography (CAT) scan: Type of scanning that adds X-ray images with the aid of a computer to generate cross-sectional views of an internal organ or bodily tissues. In dementia cases, CAT scans of the brain can be used to support a diagnosis.

confabulation: The production of fabricated, distorted or misinterpreted memories about oneself or the world without the conscious intention to deceive.

confusion: The state of being unable to think clearly, feeling disoriented or having difficulty focusing, making decisions or remembering.

corticospinal: Of or relating to the cerebral cortex and the spinal cord.

-D-

decision-making: The act of selecting a logical choice from available options.

deep brain stimulation (DBS): Surgical procedure that is effective in treating Parkinson's disease. The surgery includes the implantation of permanent electrodes in various parts of the brain through which continuous pulses of electricity are given to control the symptoms of Parkinson's disease.

deficits: Physical and/or cognitive skills or abilities that a person has lost, has difficulty with, or can no longer perform due to his or her dementia.

defining LBD symptom: A symptom used to help diagnose dementia with Lewy bodies (DLB) and Parkinson's disease dementia (PDD).

dehydration: A harmful reduction in the amount of water in the body.

delusions: False, often paranoid, beliefs that can appear alone or accompany dreams, hallucinations or actual events. Typical delusions include those of persecution, grandeur, control or misidentification.

delusions, misidentification: Delusional belief that real people or one's own home are replaced by impostors, or that the mirror image of one's self is another person. *(See Capgras syndrome)*

delusions, systemized: Delusions built into complicated dramas that can often last over time.

dementia care, palliative: Care that focuses on comfort, peace and the relief of pain and suffering rather than maintaining skills or extending life.

dementia care, proactive: Care that focuses on helping a patient use their remaining skills to maintain independence and improve quality of life..

dementia with Lewy bodies (DLB): A Lewy body dementia, where the cognitive dysfunctions precede motor dysfunctions. Symptoms include cognitive, perceptual, sleep and autonomic dysfunctions. Closely related to Parkinson's disease with dementia. (PDD). May also be called diffuse Lewy body disease, cortical Lewy body disease, dementia with Lewy body or Lewy body variant of Alzheimer's disease.

dementia: Impairment of two or more cognitive abilities. Alzheimer's disease is the most common cause of dementia; LBD and vascular dementia are the next most common. Other causes are brain injury, brain tumors, toxicity, encephalitis, meningitis, fronto-temporal lobe dementia, syphilis and thyroid disease.

depression, major: Disease that interferes with the ability to work, sleep, eat and enjoy once pleasurable activities. Often includes suicidal thoughts. (See depression.)

depression: Depressive illness involving the body, mood and thoughts. Symptoms include a loss of interests, low self-esteem, feelings of helplessness and hopelessness, poor appetite and weight loss. Can be organic (disease related) or situational. See also major depression.

Desyrel (trazodone hydrochloride): A Non-SSRI antidepressant that allows more serotonin to stimulate the nerves in the brain.

disinhibition: A loss of inhibition due to brain damage, resulting in disregard of social constraints, tactlessness, rudeness and impulsiveness and poor risk assessment.

distraction: Something that draws the patient's attention away from the present behavior.

dizziness: Painless head discomfort with many possible causes. Also called lightheadedness, unsteadiness and vertigo. Can be the result of a lack of oxygen to the brain. (See orthostatic hypotension.)

donepezil hydrochloride: See Aricept.

dopamine: An amino acid that acts as a neurotransmitter in the midbrain where it facilitates mobility.

drug sensitivity: The reaction to a normal dose as though it were an overdose. Varies greatly with each individual and each drug. (See Lewy sensitivity.)

drug, acetylcholinesterase inhibitors (AChEIs): See drug, cholinesterase inhibitors.

drug, antianxiety: (aka: tranquilizers): Drug used to treat anxiety, agitation and nervousness and as a muscle relaxant. Most are benzodiazepines and poor choices for use with LBD. Examples: Valium, Klonopin, Atarax *drug, anticholinergic:* (anti-koh-luh-nur-jik) One that impairs or weakens acetylcholine. Includes muscle relaxants, anti-anxiety drugs, sedatives and antipsychotics. Most are Lewy-sensitive.

drug, anticonvulsant: AKA: antiepileptic, or antiseizure drug. Used to control seizures (convulsions) by reducing nerve signals in the brain. May also be used to treat depression or restless leg syndrome. (Neurontin, Tegretol)

drug, antidepressant: Used to reduce depression. (Celexa, Desyrel, Paxil, Prozac and Zoloft)

drug, antidopaminergic: (anti-doh-puh-mi-nur-jik) One that impairs or weakens dopamine. Includes most dementia drugs.

drug, antipsychotics: Drugs approved for treating psychotic symptoms such as *hallucinations*, *delusions, agitation* and panic attacks in psychiatric diseases such as schizophrenia and often used "off label" with dementia.

drug, atypical antipsychotic: Second generation antipsychotics that use a different action than traditional antipsychotics and are therefore sometimes safer for LBD patients. Any use is still off-label. (Seroquel, Risperdal, Zyprexa)

drug, benzodiazepine: A family of drugs including most antianxiety drugs that work in the central nervous system. They are contraindicated for use with LBD due to the possibility of extreme drug sensitivity reactions with motor-related symptoms, loss of cognitive functions and/or muscle rigidity.

drug, cholinesterase inhibitors (ChEIs): Medication that inhibits the enzymes that convert acetylcholine into other chemicals, thus increasing the level of acetylcholine in the brain. Pro: Can decrease confusion, cognitive fluctuations and other LBD symptoms such as agitation and hallucinations. Con: often have severe gastrointestinal side effects. (Aricept, Exelon, Razadyne)

drug, Lewy sensitive: A drug known to trigger Lewy sensitivity in some patients. Includes most antipsychotics, anti-anxiety drugs, sedatives and anticholinergics. (See drug sensitivity)

213

drug, psychostimulant: Used to increase psychomotor activity. Can improve concentration and impulse control in attention deficit hyperactivity disorder. Many are addictive. (See Provigil.)

drug, sedative hypnotic: Drugs used to reduce tension, relieve anxiety and induce calm (sedative effect) or to induce sleep (hypnotic effect). Most of these drugs exert a quieting or calming effect at low doses and a sleep-inducing effect in larger doses. Due to their effect on the central nervous system, these drugs are not usually recommended for use with LBD. (Lunesta, Restoril, Seconal)

drug, selective serotonin reuptake inhibitor (SSRI): A class of antidepressant medications used to treat depression, panic attacks and other anxiety disorders. They restore the balance of neurotransmitters in the brain, thereby improving mood and feeling of well-being, without depleting acetylcholine. (Celexa, Paxil, Prozac, Zoloft)

drug, traditional antipsychotic: (aka: neuroleptics) First generation antipsychotics, seldom used anymore except in emergency rooms and hospice. (Haldol)

dry mouth: Condition of not having enough saliva to keep the mouth wet, caused by inadequately functioning salivary glands. A common drug side effect.

durable power of attorney: Type of advance medical directive in which legal documents provide the power of attorney to another person in the case of an incapacitating medical condition.

dyskinesia: Abnormal muscle movements which can occur as a side effect of certain medications such as Levodopa and antipsychotic drugs.

dysphagia: Difficulty in swallowing.

dysphasia: Speech impairment due to difficulty controlling the muscles used for speech. Sometimes considered a milder form of aphasia.

dysphoria: Anxiety.

dyspnea: Difficult or labored breathing; shortness of breath.

dyspraxia: Impaired or painful function of any organ of the body.

dystonia: Involuntary movements and prolonged muscle contraction, resulting in twisting body motions, tremor and abnormal posture. These movements may involve the entire body or only an isolated area.

-E-

elder law attorney: Attorney who practices in the area of elder law which focuses on issues typically affecting older adults.

empathy: Being able to understand and share the feelings of another.

end stage: Last phase in the course of a progressive disease.

environmental: In the air, water or food.

euphoria: Persistent and unreasonable sense of well-being.

excessive daytime sleep (EDS): (Also called excessive daytime somnolence) Persistent sleepiness and often a general lack of energy, during the day after apparently adequate or even prolonged nighttime sleep.

excitatory system: The portion of the autonomic nervous system responsible for speeding up organ activity. LBD tends to interfere with this activity, thus increasing organ inefficiency.

executive functions: Abilities used in thinking. Includes reasoning, problem solving, judgment, learning, planning, decision making, sequencing, prioritizing and generalizing.

Exelon (rivastigmine): A cholinesterase inhibitor. The Exelon skin patch bypasses the gastro-intestinal tract to reduce GI side-effects.

exercise: Activity requiring physical effort.

-F-

facial affect: The expression that shows on one's face.

familial: Tending to occur more often in family members than expected by chance alone. A familial disease may be genetic or environmental.

familiarity: Provides security because a patient knows what to expect.

fecal impaction: A large, hard mass of stool stuck in the colon or rectum that can't be pushed out.

Federal Drug Administration (FDA): The section of government that oversees the manufacturing and distribution of food and drugs.

festination: Walking in rapid, short, shuffling steps.

flexibility: The ability to switch from one concept to another, to review the evidence and change your mind.

Florinef (fludrocortisone acetate): Medication used to treat orthostatic hypotension.

fluctuating cognition: Periods of increased arousal, attention and cognition occurring over minutes to hours alternating with periods of much more severe sleepiness, confusion, disorientation and forgetfulness. A defining LBD symptom.

fludrocortisone acetate: See Florinef.

fluoxetine hydrochloride: See Prozac.

flushing: An involuntary response of the nervous system leading to a temporary widening of the capillaries of the involved skin. Usually caused by excitement, exercise, fever, or embarrassment but can also be caused by medications that widen the capillaries, such as niacin.

Foley catheter: Flexible plastic tube (catheter) inserted into the bladder to provide drainage of urine on a continuous basis.

Fronto-temporal dementia (FTD): Also called Pick's disease. Form of dementia caused by a shrinkage of the frontal and temporal lobes of the brain. Can be hereditary. It is characterized by a slowly progressive deterioration of social skills and changes in personality leading to impairment of intellect, memory and language. Results in behavior problems, including severe apathy and lack of compassion or empathy.

-G-

gabapentin: See Neurontin.

gait: Manner of walking. People with dementia often have reduced gait, meaning their ability to lift their feet as they walk has diminished.

galantamine hydrobromide: See Razadyne.

gastrointestinal (GI) tract: The part of the digestive system that includes the stomach, small and large intestines.

gene: The basic unit by which genetic information is passed from parent to offspring.

generic drug: A drug created to be the same as an existing approved brand-name drug, Produced and distributed without patent protection, these drugs are usually much less expensive than their brand name forerunners.

generic: The chemical name of a drug.

genetic: Inherited.

geriatric: Pertaining to the elderly.

gerontology: Study of the aging process including physical, mental and social changes. A gerontologist is a psychologist with a master's degree or doctorate in gerontology.

glutamate: A neurotransmitter that facilitates cognitive and perceptive functions.

Good Times: The times when a patient is more alert and aware as compared to the Bad Times. (See cognitive fluctuations.)

guardian: Individual appointed by the courts who is authorized to make legal and financial decisions for another individual.

-H-

Haldol: Trade name for haloperidol: Traditional antipsychotic drug. Particularly dangerous for LBD patients.

hallucination: A sensory experience in which a person experiences something unreal as very real. Hallucinations can also be auditory (hearing), gustatory (taste), kinesthetic (body movement) Lilliputian (people and things appearing smaller than normal), musical (auditory hallucination concerning music), olfactory (smell) or tactile (touch).

healthy diet: A diet that includes those nutrients needed to maintain health, energy and happiness.

here and now: the present, with no reference to past or present.

heredity: Genetic transmission from parent to child.

home health care: Provision of skilled health care and custodial health aides services in the home on a part-time basis for the treatment of an illness or injury.

hospice: Program or facility that provides palliative care for people who are near the end of life and for their families.

hypokinesia: Abnormal decrease in muscular movement.

hyposmia: loss of the sense of smell.

-I-

idiopathic: Of unknown cause.

illusion: A misinterpreted perception of a sensory experience.

impulse control: The ability to pick and choose how to respond to a feeling or an event.

incontinence: Inability to control excretions. Urinary incontinence is the inability to keep urine in the bladder. Fecal incontinence is the inability to retain feces in the rectum.

inhibitory system: The portion of the autonomic nervous system responsible for inhibiting, or slowing down organ activity. LBD tends to increase this function, slowing down organ activity even more.

insomnia: Difficulty falling asleep, difficulty returning to sleep, waking up too soon or unrefreshing sleep.

instrumental activities of daily living (IADLs): Secondary level of activities during daily living such as cooking, writing and driving.

irritability: Quality or state of being irritable; testiness or petulance.

-J-

judgment: The process of reviewing the available information and making a decision.

-K-

Klonopin (clonazepam): A benzodiazipine-based anti-anxiety drug used to treat Active Dreams. Mildly anticholinergic.

-L-

levodopa/carbidopa: See Sinemet.

levodopa: Generic drug used together with carbidopa to treat the symptoms of Parkinson's disease. Used alone, it may cause adverse side effects. (See Sinemet.)

Lewy bodies: Misfolded alpha-synuclein proteins that clump loosely together in neurons, expand and spread. (See alpha-synuclein and protein, misfolded.)

Lewy body dementia (LBD). Dementia caused by Lewy bodies in the brain. Includes both dementia with Lewy bodies (DLB) and Parkinson's disease with dementia. (PDD). Closely related to Parkinson's disease and multiple system atrophy (MSA).

Lewy sensitivity: Drug sensitivity specific to LBD. (see drug sensitivity.)

listening: A more successful response than explaining.

living will: Legal document in which the signer requests not to be kept alive by medical life-support or life prolonging systems in the event of a terminal illness.

long-term care (LTC): Personal care services given at home or in a skilled nursing facility for people with chronic disabilities and lengthy illnesses. Medicare does not generally cover long-term care.

long-term care facility (LTCF): Facility that provides rehabilitative, restorative and/or ongoing skilled nursing care to patients or residents in need of assistance with activities of daily living.

long-term care ombudsman: advocate who resolves disputes between residents of skilled nursing facilities or assisted living care facilities and the facility management. This individual also works to inform residents and their family members of their rights and protections while residing in a facility.

-M-

magnetic resonance imaging (MRI): Radiology technique designed to image internal structures of the body using magnetism, radio waves and a computer to produce the images of body structures.

mask-like face: Facial affect with little or no sense of animation. Seen in Parkinson's disease.

Medicaid: State programs of public assistance to persons regardless of age whose income and resources are insufficient to pay for health care. The United States federal government provides matching funds to state Medicaid programs.

Medicare: US government's health insurance program for individuals 65 years of age or older, certain younger people with specific disabilities or end-stage renal disease.

melatonin: A hormone that regulates the body's sleep cycle. Used to treat sleep disorders such as Active Dreams and insomnia.

memantine hydrochloride: See Namenda.

memory span: Number of items, usually words or numbers that a person can retain and recall. Memory span is a test of short-term memory function. The average span for normal adults is seven.

memory, long term: Permanently stores, manages and retrieves information for later use. Items of information stored as long-term memory may be available for a lifetime.

memory, short term: Temporarily stores information about recent events and sensory data and holds programs or data currently in use.

memory, working: An area of high-speed memory used to out carry out complex cognitive tasks such as learning, reasoning and comprehension.

memory: Ability or process of storing, encoding and retrieving information.

mental stimulation: Anything that stimulates the brain and increases its mental reserves.

midodrine: See ProAmatine.

Mini Mental State Exam (MMSE): Exam for determining the mental status of a person. Performed by a health care professional. The test measures a person's basic cognitive skills, such as short-term memory, long-term memory, orientation, writing and language.

Mirapex (pramipexole): Medication used to treat Parkinson's disease to provide replacement for the neurotransmitter dopamine.

mobility: The ability to move.

modafinil: See Provigil.

multiple system atrophy (MSA): A progressive neurodegenerative disorder characterized by a combination of symptoms that affect both the autonomic nervous system and movement.

muscle atonia: restrained muscle activity, except middle ear muscle activity and eye movement.

-N-

Namenda (memantine hydrochloride): Dementia drug. Works with the neurotransmitter glutamate. Seldom used alone with LBD but useful as an adjunct to cholinesterase inhibitors.

National Institute of Health (NIH): US health agency devoted to medical research. It consists of 20 plus separate Institutes and Centers including NIMH, NINDS and NIA.

National Institute of Neurological Disorders and Stroke (NINDS): A NIH institute with the mission of researching nervous system disorders for causes, prevention, diagnosis and treatment.

National Institute on Aging (NIA): A NIH institute with the mission of researching the biomedical, social and behavioral aspects of the aging processes to promote prevention of age related diseases and disabilities for a better quality of life for the elderly.

nerves: Bundles of neuron fibers that make up a network of information pathways and use chemical and electrical signals to transmit sensory and motor information from one body part to another.

neurodegenerative: Relating to or characterized by degeneration of nervous tissue.

neuroleptic sensitivity: Reaction to a neuroleptic (antipsychotic) drug, causing side-effects including increased confusion, rigidity, immobility and an inability to perform tasks or to communicate. May or may not be permanent. Is present in at least 50% of LBD patients; with use of traditional antipsychotic drugs increasing morbidity 2-3 fold.

neurological: Having to do with the nerves or the nervous system, the brain, the spinal cord and nerves.

neurologist: A physician who specializes in the diagnosis and treatment of disorders of the nervous system.

neurology: Medical specialty concerned with the diagnosis and treatment of disorders of the nervous system.

neuron: Nerve cell that sends and receives electrical signals over long distances within the body.

Neurontin (gabapentin): Anticonvulsive drug used to treat Restless Leg Syndrome.

neuropathologist: A pathologist who specializes in the diagnosis of diseases of the brain and nervous system by microscopic examination of the tissue and other means.

neuropathy: Disease or dysfunction of one or more peripheral nerves, typically causing numbness or weakness.

neuropsychiatrist: A psychiatrist who specializes in neurology.

neuropsychological testing: Assessment of cognitive abilities such as memory, attention, orientation to time and place, use of language, ability to carry out various tasks and follow instructions.

neuropsychologist: A psychologist who has completed special training in neurology and who specializes in diagnosing and treating neurological illnesses using a predominantly medical approach.

neurotransmitter: A chemical messenger, a compound that transmits an impulse from a nerve cell to another nerve, muscle, organ or other tissue.

nightmares: Dream arousing feelings of intense fear, horror or distress.

nurse: A person trained, licensed or skilled in nursing.

nurse practitioner (NP): Registered nurse who has completed an advanced training program in some medical specialty, can function as a primary direct provider of health care and can prescribe medications.

nurse, licensed practical (LPN) or licensed vocational (LVN): Nurse who has completed a one- or two-year training program in health care and earned a state license. LPNs provide direct patient care for people with chronic illness, in nursing homes, hospitals and home settings. They assist RNs in caring for patients.

nurse, registered (RN): Nurse who has completed a two- to four-year degree program in nursing. RNs provide direct patient care and supervision of other care staff. RNs may further specialize in a particular area.

nursing assistant, certified (CNA): Person who has completed a brief health-care training program and has been certified by a state agency. CNAs provide support services for RNs and LPNs. Also known as nursing aid or orderly when uncertified.

nursing home: Residential facility for persons with chronic illness or disability, particularly older people who have mobility and eating problems. Also called a convalescent home, long-term care facility or a skilled nursing facility.

-O-

occupational therapist (OT): Works with anyone who has a permanent or temporary impairment in their physical or mental functioning. The aim of occupational therapy is to help the client to perform daily tasks in their living and working environments and to assist them to develop the skills to live independent, satisfying and productive lives.

off-label: Used in a way not approved by the Federal Drug Administration.

olanzapine: See Zyprexa.

orthostatic hypotension (OH): AKA low blood pressure on rising. Temporary lowering of blood pressure (hypotension) due usually to suddenly standing up (orthostatic). The change in position causes a temporary reduction in blood flow and therefore a shortage of oxygen to the brain. This leads to lightheadedness and, sometimes, syncope.

-P-

paradoxical reaction: A reaction opposite to that expected, usually resulting in an increase rather than decrease of the treated symptom.

paranoia: Suspiciousness or mistrust exhibited by dementia patients as their memory becomes worse. For example, a patient misplaces a possession but believes it has been stolen.

parasympathetic nervous system: Part of the autonomic nervous system that slows the heart rate, increases intestinal and gland activity and relaxes sphincter muscles.

Parkinson's disease (PD): Slowly progressive neurological disease characterized by a fixed inexpressive face, a tremor at rest, slowing of voluntary movements, a gait with short accelerating steps, peculiar posture and muscle weakness, caused by degeneration of an area of the brain called the basal ganglia and by low production of the neurotransmitter dopamine.

parkinsonian symptoms: Movement dysfunctions in an individual who may or may not be diagnosed with Parkinson's.

parkinsonism: A collective name for motor and mobility symptoms such as those that show up in Parkinson's but also in other diseases including DLB. May be caused by drugs used to treat other symptoms.

paroxetine: See Paxil.

Paxil: (paroxetine): One of the SSRI antidepressants. See selective serotonin reuptake inhibitor.

perception: The interpretation of information delivered to the brain by the senses.

physical therapy (PT): Branch of rehabilitative health that uses specially designed exercises and equipment to help patients regain or improve their physical abilities. A physical therapist is a person trained and certified to provide these services.

physician assistant (PA): Mid-level medical practitioner who works under the supervision of a licensed doctor (an MD) or osteopathic physician (a DO).

physician, family, general or primary: Medical doctor who provides continuing and comprehensive health care for the individual and family. Usually the first physician a patient sees before being referred to a specific specialist.

physician: Person trained in the art of healing and is also referred to as a medical doctor or MD.

plaques: Lesions of brain tissue found along with tangles in Alzheimer's disease.

positron emission tomography (PET) scan: Highly specialized imaging technique that uses short-lived radioactive substances to produce three-dimensional colored images (PET scans) of metabolic activity or body functions. The PET scan has been used to assess adult dementia.

postural instability: Inability to maintain a correct posture in either a standing or sitting position. A Parkinson's symptom.

pramipexole: See Mirapex.

ProAmatine (midodrine): Medication which can be used to treat orthostatic hypotension.

problem solving: The process of working through the details of a problem to reach a solution.

progressive decline: Ongoing, continually getting worse.

progressive supranuclear palsy (PSP): Neurologic disorder of unknown origin that gradually destroys cells in many areas of the brain, leading to serious and permanent problems with the control of gait and balance. Patients also often show alterations of mood and behavior, including depression, apathy and dementia.

progressive: Increasing in scope or severity; advancing, going forward.

propulsive gait: Disturbance of gait; during walking, steps become faster and faster with progressively shorter steps that pass from a walking to a running pace and may precipitate falling forward.

protein, misfolded: A protein that has been changed or damaged, so that it does something else instead of its intended task.

protein: The body's building block, composed of amino acids and used for the structure, function and regulation of the body's cells, tissues and organs.

Provigil (modafinil): Psychostimulant drug used to treat excessive daytime sleepiness or problems with breathing while asleep. May also improve alertness in dementia patients. Considered less addictive than other psychostimulants.

Prozac (fluoxetine hydrochloride): A SSRI antidepressant. (See selective serotonin reuptake inhibitors.)

psychiatry: Medical specialty concerned with the prevention, diagnosis and treatment of mental illness. A psychiatrist is a physician who specializes in psychiatry.

psychology: Study of the mind and mental processes, especially in relation to behavior. A psychologist is a person with a masters or doctorate in psychology who uses talk or behavioral therapy as treatment. They cannot prescribe medication but usually work closely with a physician or psychiatrist who can.

psychomotor: Of or relating to movement or muscular activity associated with mental processes.

psychopharmacology: Management of psychiatric illness using medication such as antidepressants, antipsychotics, anti-anxiety drugs and more.

psychosis: Mental illness that markedly interferes with a person's capacity to meet life's everyday demands. Symptoms can include hallucinations, paranoia and delusional thoughts.

-Q-

quetiapine: See Seroquel.

-R-

Razadyne (galantamine hydrobromide): Formerly known as Reminyl. An cholinesterase inhibitor used to treat mild or moderate dementia. See cholinesterase inhibitor.

reaction: Acting without thought.

reality: A person's world view, a belief not open to negotiation.

reasoning: The process of forming logical decisions, judgments or inferences based on available information such as facts, theories or intuition.

receptor: Structure on the surface of a nerve cell (or inside a cell) that receives and responds to stimuli.

reduplicative paramnesia: A delusional belief that a place or location has been duplicated, existing in two or more places simultaneously, or that it has been 'relocated' to another site.

rehabilitation: The process of helping an injured or ill person restore lost skills and regain or retain maximum self-sufficiency.

REM (rapid eye movement) sleep: Portion of sleep when there are rapid eye movements. Dreams occur during REM sleep. (see REM sleep behavior disorder)

REM sleep behavior disorder (RBD): AKA Active Dreams. A Lewy body disorder and a defining LBD symptom. Loss of normal muscle atonia (paralysis) during REM sleep allows physical acting out of one's dreams.

respite program: Program that enables a person to take needed breaks from being a care partner.

response: A thought out action.

restless leg syndrome (RLS): Uncontrollable urge to move legs to relieve uncomfortable sensations such a creeping, tingling, twitching, throbbing or prickling. The sensations typically become more noticeable with rest (sitting or lying down) and ease with motion.

retropulsion: Tendency to fall or move backwards.

rigidity: Increased muscle tone in neck, arms or legs.

*Risperdal (*risperidone): An atypical antipsychotic drug sometimes used off-label to treat dementia-related behaviors.

risperidone: See Risperdal.

rivastigmine: See Exelon.

routine: A sequence of activities that doesn't vary or change.

-S-

security: The state of feeling safe and in control.

sedative hypnotic drug: Acts to assist sleep by depressing the central nervous system. May cause serious side effects for LBD patients. Often very addictive. (Ambien, Lunesta)

Seroquel (quetiapine): Atypical antipsychotic. Insomnia can also be treated with this drug. Often the antipsychotic of choice for LBD patients.

sertraline: See Zoloft.

Showtime: When a LBD patient acts "normal" for a limited time in the presence of someone other than their caregiver. See fluctuating cognition, Bad Times and Good Times.

Sinemet (carbidopa/levodopa): A drug used to control motor dysfunctions.

Sinemet (levodopa/carbidopa): A drug used to treat Parkinson's symptoms. The levodopa treats the symptoms and carbidopa decreases levodopa's side effects.

Single Photon Emission Computed Tomography scan (SPECT scan): An imaging procedure using radioactive tracers in which a gamma camera rotates around the patient and takes pictures from many angles, which a computer then uses to form a tomographic (cross-sectional) image.

skilled nursing facility (SNF): Institution providing persons 65+ years of age (and younger disabled persons) with daily skilled nursing care, rehabilitation and other medical services.

sleep apnea: Temporary stoppage of breathing during sleep, often resulting in daytime sleepiness. Most likely due to the relaxation of throat muscles.

socialization: Interacting with other people, one of the most important human needs.

spatial disorientation: Inability to determine one's position, location and motion relative to their environment.

speak to the emotion: Voicing the emotion being expressed by the patient.

spinal cord: The cord of nervous tissue that extends from the brain lengthwise along the back in the spinal canal and serves as a center for initiating and coordinating many reflex acts.

stages: Course of a disease progression defined by levels or periods of severity: early, mild, moderate, moderately severe and severe.

substantia nigra: Layer of large pigmented nerve cells in the mid-brain that produce dopamine and whose destruction is associated with Parkinson's disease.

sympathetic nervous system: Part of the autonomic nervous system which accelerates the heart rate, constricts blood vessels and raises blood pressure.

synapse: Point of connection (or communication) between two nerve cells.

syncope: Partial or complete loss of consciousness caused by a fall in blood pressure and a resultant lack of oxygen in the brain. Recovery is spontaneous.

-T-

tangles: Twisted fibers that build up around nerve cells of patients with Alzheimer's disease. (plaques)

taste buds: sensory sites in the mouth that identify sweet, salty, sour, bitter and savory.

Tegretol (carbamazepine): Anticonvulsant sometimes used to treat mental illness, depression, restless leg syndrome. (Neurontin)

thinking error: A thought that has not been filtered by a person's complex thinking abilities, resulting in misinformation and delusions.

toxins: Substances known to be damaging to the body.

trazodone hydrochloride: See Desyrel.

tremor: Any abnormal repetitive shaking, often involving the fingers, arms or legs.

tremor, intentional: AKA active or essential tremor. Tremor occurring when a person attempts voluntary movement such as writing or lifting a cup.

tremor, resting: AKA passive tremor. Tremor that occurs when the body is at rest and diminishes or stops during voluntary movement.

-U--V-

vascular dementia (VaD): Common form of dementia due to cerebrovascular disease, caused by a series of small strokes, each of which causes a small loss of cognitive functions.

verbal blocking: Difficulty in expressing full sentences and losing track of one's thoughts.

visual perceptual abilities: Vision-related perceptual abilities such as hand-eye coordination, depth perception and other vision-related tasks which are often damaged by LBD.

visuospatial function: Cognitive function related to the combination of visual and spatial awareness. Also called hand-eye coordination.

-W-

wanting to go home: Wanting to feel "normal."

word recall difficulties: Difficulty remembering a specific word--"it's on the tip of my tongue" syndrome."

word substitution: Substituting another word, often an inappropriate one, for the one a person means.

-X -Y-

-Z-

Zoloft (sertraline): SSRI antidepressant used to treat depression, panic attacks and other anxiety type disorders. See selective serotonin reuptake inhibitors.

zolpidem tartrate: See Ambien.

Zyprexa (olanzapine): Atypical antipsychotic which has not been shown to be safe or effective treatment for elderly people with dementia. (See antipsychotic, atypical.)

Acronyms

AAN	American Academy of Neurology
ACh-E	acetylcholine esterase
AChEIs	acetylcholinesterase inhibitors
ACh-R	acetylcholine receptors
AD	Alzheimer's disease
ADAS-Cog	Alzheimer's disease assessment scale-cognitive subscale
ADC	Alzheimer's Disease Center
ADEAR	Alzheimer's Disease Education and Referral Center
ADRC	Alzheimer's Disease Research Center
ADRDA	Alzheimer's Disease and Related Disorders Association
ALF	assisted living facility
ADL	activities of daily living (also see IADL)
ANS	autonomic nervous system (also see S-ANS and P-ANS)
AS	alpha-synuclein
BNT	Boston naming test
BS	bachelor of science degree
CAMCOG	Cambridge Mental Disorders of the Elderly Examination
CANTAB	Cambridge Neuropsychological Test Automated Battery
CAT	Computerized Axial Tomography
CBD	corticobasal degeneration
CBD	Cannabidiol (medical marijuana component)
CDC	Center for Disease Control (and prevention)
CDR	clinical dementia rating (scale)
CG	caregiver
ChAT	cortical choline acetyltransferase
ChEIs	cholinesterase inhibitors
CJD	Creutzfeldt-Jakob disease (prion disease)
CLBD	(See LBD)
CMS	Center for Medicare and Medicaid Services (US Govt Agency)
CNA	certified nursing aid

CNS	central nervous system
CPR	cardiopulmonary resuscitation
CSH	carotid sinus hypersensitivity
CSS	carotid sinus syndrome
CT	computed tomography (scan)
CVD	cerebrovascular disease
CVLT	California Verbal Learning Test (long-delay recall, percent retained)
DA	dopamine
DAT	dopamine active transporter
DBS	deep brain stimulation
DLB	dementia with Lewy bodies
DLBD	diffuse Lewy body dementia
DNR	do not resuscitate
DRS	dementia rating scale
DSM	Diagnostic and Statistical Manual of Mental Disorders
DSM-IV	DSM 4th Version
DSM-5	DSM 5th Version
ECG	electrocardiogram
ECT	electroconvulsive therapy
EEG	electroencephalogram
EKG	(see ECG)
EPS	extrapyramidal motor symptoms
EOG	electro-oculogram
ET	essential tremor
FDA	federal drug administration
FRCP	Fellow of the Royal College of Physicians
FTD	frontotemporal dementia (or Pick's disease)
FTDP-17	frontotemportal dementia with parkinsonism related to chromosome 17
HD	Huntington's disease
HVLT	Hopkins verbal learning test
IADL	instrumental activities of daily living
IBS	irritable bowel syndrome

ICD	International Classification of Disease (World Health Organization)
ICD-9	ICD Symptom Checklist for Mental Disorders, Ver. 9
ICD-10	ICD Symptom Checklist for Mental Disorders, Ver. 10
IHC	immunohistochemistry
IU	international unit of drug
IV	1) intravenous; 2) roman numeral 4 as in 4th edition
LB	Lewy bodies
LBD	Lewy body dementia, also known as:
	Lewy body disease
	diffuse Lewy body disease
	cortical Lewy body disease
LBDA	Lewy Body Dementia Association, Inc.
LBV	Lewy body variant
LCPC	licensed clinical counselor
LNs	Lewy neuritis
LPN	licensed practical nurse
LTC	long-term care
LTCF	long-term care facility
LTHC	long-term health care
LVN	licensed vocational nurse
MAOI	monoamine oxidase inhibitor antidepressants
MCI	mild cognitive impairment
MD	doctor of medicine
MG	myasthenia gravis (auto-immune disease)
MID	multi-infarct dementia
MIBG	iodine-131-meta-iodobenzylguanidine
MMSE	mini mental state examination
MPH	Master of Public Health (degree)
MRI	magnetic resonance imaging
MRS	magnetic resonance spectroscopy
MSA	multiple system atrophy
MS	1) multiple sclerosis; 2) master of science degree
NAChR	nicotinic acetylcholine receptors

NCVI	neurocardiovascular instability
NFT	neurofibrillary tangles
NIA	National Institute of Aging
NIA-RI	National Institute of Aging and Reagan Institute
NIH	National Institute of Health
NIMH	National Institute of Mental Health
NINDS	National Institute of Neurological Disorders and Strokes
NMS	neuroleptic malignant syndrome
NP	nurse practitioner
NPF	National Parkinson's Foundation
NPI	Neuropsychiatric Inventory
NFT	neurofibrillary tangles
OH	orthostatic hypotension
OSA	obstructive sleep apnea
OT	occupational therapist
OTC	over the counter medication (non-prescription)
PA	physician assistant
PAF	pure autonomic failure
P-ANS	parasympathic part of the ANS
PD	Parkinson's disease
PDD	Parkinson's disease with dementia
PDF	Parkinson's Disease Foundation
PET	positron emission tomography (scan)
PhD	doctoral research degree
PIGD	postural instability and gait disorder (or difficulty)
PKAN	pantothenate kinase deficiency
PLM	periodic limb movement
PPI	prepulse inhibition
PSP	progressive supranuclear palsy
PT	physical therapy
RBD	REM sleep behavioral disorder
REM	rapid eye movement
RLS	restless leg syndrome
RN	registered nurse

RT	resting tremor
S-ANS	sympathetic part of the ANS
SCNA	alpha-synuclein gene
SDLT	senile dementia of Lewy body type (See LBD)
SIVD	subcortical ischemic vascular dementia
SNF	skilled nursing facility
SPECT	single-photon emission computed tomography
SSRI	selective serotonin reuptake inhibitors
TD	tardive dyskinesia
TIA	transient ischemic attack (non-damaging warning stroke)
UPDRS	unified Parkinson's disease rating scale
VA	Veterans Affairs
Vad	vascular dementia
VCD	vascular cognitive disorder
VCJD	variant of CJD (believed to be human form of BSE "mad cow disease")
VCI	vascular cognitive impairment
VCI-ND	vascular cognitive impairment no dementia
VH	visual hallucinations

References

You can find a list of the digital references used in this book at www.lbdtools.com/rcbook.html. (Please be aware that over time, some links disappear.)

[1] **National Institutes of Health.** Dementia Information Page. NINDS. https://www.ninds.nih.gov/Disorders/All-Disorders/Dementia-Information-Page.

[2] **Melao A**. (2018) UNS' Investigational Vaccine UB-312 Holds Potential to Prevent Parkinson's, Other Neurological Diseases, Data Show. Parkinson's News Today. November 16, 2018. https://parkinsonsnewstoday.com/2018/11/16/vaccine-ub-312-may-prevent-parkinsons-other-diseases-data-show/

[3] **Rogers M.**(2018) Estrogen's Benefit Tied to Age: Good for the Young, Bad for the Old. Alzheimer's Association International Conference 2018. Chicago, Illinois 22 – 26 July 2018. https://www.alzforum.org/news/conference-coverage/estrogens-benefit-tied-age-good-young-bad-old#tools

[4] Hara Y. (2017) New Debate On Hormone Replacement Therapy And Dementia Risk. March 22, 2017.Cognitive Vitality. Alzheimer's Drug Discovery Foundation. https://www.alzdiscovery.org/cognitive-vitality/blog/new-debate-on-hormone-replacement-therapy-and-dementia-risk

[5] **IOS Press.** (2018, March 26). Neuroscientists say daily ibuprofen can prevent Alzheimer's disease. Science Daily. March 26, 2018. www.sciencedaily.com/releases/2018/03/180326140239.htm

[6] Cannell J. (2018) Alzheimer's disease. Vitamin D council.January 26, 2018. https://www.vitamindcouncil.org/health-conditions/alzheimers-disease/#.XWPheONKiM8

[7] Burckhardt M, et. al. (2016) Omega-3 fatty acids for the treatment of dementia. Cochrane. https://www.cochrane.org/CD009002/DEMENTIA_omega-3-fatty-acids-treatment-dementia

[8] **Caselli R.** (2008) Alzheimer's Disease: Diagnosis and Treatment. Presented May 30, 2008, at the Arizona Alzheimer'sConsortium 2008 Annual Conference.

[9] **Marquez J**. (2018) What's Really Giving You Alzheimer's. AARP, September 25, 2018. https://www.aarp.org/health/dementia/info-2018/dementia-risk-factors.html

[10] **Ingram I**. (2018) Parkinson, Depression Meds Tied to Dementia Risk. MedPage Today. April 25, 2018. https://www.medpagetoday.com/neurology/dementia/72545

[11] **Costa S.** (2015) Living with Lewy Body Dementia. U.S. News. Sept. 22, 2015. https://health.usnews.com/health-news/patient-advice/articles/2015/09/22/living-with-lewy-body-dementia

[12] **Whitworth H and J**. Responsive Dementia Care: Fewer Behaviors Fewer Drugs. Oleander Books, 2018. http://www.responsivedementiacare.com/

[13] **Hatfiled L**. (2016) Sleep Centers: On the Frontline for the Future of Lewy Body Dementia. Axovant Sciences, Inc. http://a360-wp-uploads.s3.amazonaws.com/wp-content/uploads/sleeprev/2017/03/RBDLewyBodyDementia1.pdf

[14] **Csukly G, et al.** (2016) "The Differentiation of Amnestic Type MCI from the Non-Amnestic Types by Structural MRI" Frontiers in aging neuroscience vol. 8 52. 30 Mar. 2016, doi:10.3389/fnagi.2016.00052. https://www.ncbi.nlm.nih.gov/pmc/articles/PMC4811920/

[15] **Hobson P and Mera J.** (1999) The detection of dementia in a community population of elderly people with Parkinson's disease by use of the CAMCOG neuropsychological test. Age and Ageing 1999; 28:39-43. The Oxford Journals: http://ageing.oxfordjournals.org/cgi/reprint/28/1/39.pdf.

[16] **McKeith, I G, et al.** (2017) Diagnosis and management of dementia with Lewy bodies: Fourth consensus report of the DLB Consortium. Neurology vol. 89(1): 88-100. https://www.ncbi.nlm.nih.gov/pmc/articles/PMC5496518/

[17] **Emre M, et al.** (2007) Clinical diagnostic criteria for dementia associated with Parkinson's disease. Movement Disorders. 2007;22(12):1689-1707.

[18] **Anonymous.** (2017) How Social Interaction Plays a Principal Role in Dementia. The Caregiver Space. Oct. 5, 2017. Unnamed guest author. https://thecaregiverspace.org/how-social-interaction-plays-a-principal-role-in-dementia/

[19] **Stern Y**. (2007) Build Your Cognitive Reserve. July 23, 2007. http://www.sharpbrains.com/blog/2007/07/23/build-your-cognitive-reserve-yaakov-stern/ .

[20] **Mizen M.** (2004) Scrapbook photo albums are therapeutic for Alzheimer'spatients/ Creative Memories, St. Cloud, MN. The Brain Injury Alliance of Oregon: http://www.biaoregon.org/docetc/pdf/conf05/Alzheimer%20Info.pdf

[21] **McKeehan N.** (2018) Is Exercise Bad For Dementia Patients? A New Study Makes Odd Claim. US Alzheimer's Drug Discovery Foundation. Cognitive Vitality. https://www.alzdiscovery.org/cognitive-vitality/blog/is-exercise-bad-for-dementia-patients

[22] **Alheimer's Australia.** (2015) What You Eat and Drink and Your Brain. Helpsheet Dementia Q&/A07. FightDementia. https://fightdementia.org.au/sites/default/files/helpsheets/Helpsheet-DementiaQandA07-WhatYouEatAndDrinkAndYourBrain_english.pdf

[23] **Lava N.** (2019) Medications for Parkinson's Disease. WebMD Medical Reference. Reviewed January 20, 2019. https://www.webmd.com/parkinsons-disease/guide/drug-treatments#1

[24] **Steinberg M and Lyketsos C.** (2012). Atypical Antipsychotic Use In Patients With Dementia: Managing Safety Concerns. The American Journal of Psychiatry, 169(9), 900–906. http://doi.org/10.1176/appi.ajp.2012.12030342

[25] **LBDA Scientific Advisory Council.** (2008) Medical Alert Card. Lewy Body Dementia Assn. and Novartis Pharmaceuticals. https://www.lbda.org/content/lbd-medical-alert-wallet-card

[26] **Muench J and Hamer A**. (2010) Adverse Effects of Antipsychotic Medications. Am Fam Physician. 2010 Mar 1;81(5):617-622. https://www.aafp.org/afp/2010/0301/p617.html

[27] **Bosely S** (2018) Some antidepressants linked to dementia risk. The Guardian, Wed 25 Apr 2018. https://www.theguardian.com/society/2018/apr/25/some-antidepressants-linked-to-dementia-risk

[28] **Flamm H.** (2018) "They Want Docile." How Nursing Homes in the United States Overmedicate People with Dementia. (2018) Human RightsWatch. https://www.hrw.org/report/2018/02/05/they-want-docile/how-nursing-homes-united-states-overmedicate-people-dementia#84ffd6

[29] **Pelak V and Brazis P.** (2007) Approach to the patient with visual hallucinations. http://www.utdonline.com/patients/content/topic.do?topicKey=~Wo CoPnIkImVTFL

[30] **Josephs K.** (2007) Capgras Syndrome and Its Relationship to Neurodegenerative Disease. Arch Neurol. 2007;64(12):1762-1766. http://archneur.jamanetwork.com/article.aspx?articleid=794900.

[31] **Marsh L.** Psychosis in Parkinson's Disease. Primary Psychiatry. 2005;12(7);56-62. http://primarypsychiatry.com/psychosis-in-parkinsonas-disease/.

[32] **Haehner A, et al.** (2011). Olfactory loss in Parkinson's disease. Parkinson's disease, 2011, 450939. doi: 10.4061/2011/450939

[33] **Po-Chi C, et al.** (2018) REM Sleep Behavior Disorder (RBD) in Dementia with Lewy Bodies (DLB) Behavioral Neurology, Volume 2018, Article ID 9421098, 10 pages, 2018. https://doi.org/10.1155/2018/9421098

[34] **LBDA.** (2015) Medication Glossary. Drug Classes And Medication. https://www.lbda.org/sites/default/files/medication_glossary_2015.pdf

35 **Smith M, et. al.** (2018) Restless Legs Syndrome (RLS). Symptoms, Self-help and Treatment Alternatives. https://www.helpguide.org/articles/sleep/restless-leg-syndrome-rls.htm

36 **U.S. National Library of Medicine.** (2019) Pramipexole. MedlinePlus. Updated 25 March 2019. https://medlineplus.gov/druginfo/meds/a697029.html

37 **Trotti L.** (2017) Quinine Treatment for RLS or Leg Cramps is Associated with Increased Mortality. NightWalkers, Summer 2017 edition. The Restless Leg Foundation blog: http://rlsfoundation.blogspot.com/2017/10/rls-quinine-update.html.

38 **Boeve B.** (2008). Update on the Diagnosis and Management of Sleep Disturbances in Dementia. Sleep medicine clinics, 3(3), 347–360. doi:10.1016/j.jsmc.2008.04.010

39 **Eres R, et al.** (2015). Anatomical differences in empathy related brain areas: A voxel-based morphometry study. April 24, 2015. XII International Conference on Cognitive Neuroscience doi: 10.3389/conf.fnhum.2015.217.00187

40 **Cowles C.** (2018) Diagnosing and Treating Apathy in Dementia. Caring for the Ages, July 1, 2018. Volume 19, Issue 7, p 12 https://doi.org/10.1016/j.carage.2018.06.019

41 **Smith M, et. al.** (2018) Depression Symptoms and Warning Signs. Helpguide.org. January, 2018. https://www.helpguide.org/articles/depression/depression-symptoms-and-warning-signs.htm

42 **Parkinsons Foundation.** (2019) Anxiety. Understanding-Parkinsons/Symptoms/Non-Movement-Symptoms/Anxiety. https://www.parkinson.org/Understanding-Parkinsons/Symptoms/Non-Movement-Symptoms/Anxiety

43 **Landos E, et al.** (2013) Dysphagia in Lewy body dementia - a clinical observational study of swallowing function by videofluoroscopic examination.BMC Neurol. 2013 Oct 7;13:140. doi: 10.1186/1471-2377-13-140.

[44] **Standford Medicine.** Orthostatic Hypotension in PD. parkinsons.stanford.edu/orthostatic_hypotension.html

[45] **Alzheimer Scotland.** (2011) Constipation & faecal impaction. IS 41 August 2011 Information Sheet. https://www.alzscot.org/assets/0000/0175/constipation-and-faecal-impaction.pdf

[46] **Merck Manual.** (2008) Intimacy and Dementia. The Merck Manual, Section 4, Chapter 63. Retrieved July 16, 2008 from the Merck Manual website: http://www.merckmanuals.com/home/older-people%E2%80%99s-health-issues/social-issues-affecting-older-people/intimacy-and-older-people.

[47] **Keren, R**. (June, 2005) Diagnosis and Management of Dementia with Lewy Bodies. Canadian Alzheimer'sDisease Review. http://www.stacommunications.com/customcomm/Back-issue_pages/Alzheimer's_Review/adPDFs/2005/june2005e/04.pdf.

[48] **Boot P, et. al.** (2013) Treatment of dementia with lewy bodies. Current treatment options in neurology, 15(6), 738–764. doi:10.1007/s11940-013-0261-6

[49] **Moore C.** (2015) How to Stop a Full Bladder From Killing Your Sleep. December 9, 2015 Cleveland Clinic. https://health.clevelandclinic.org/stop-full-bladder-killing-sleep/.

[50] **Walsh N.** (2003) Growing evidence: cranberry juice tied to lower UTI risk. http://www.thefreelibrary.com/Growing+evidence%3a+cranberry+juice+tied+to+lower+UTI+risk.-a0107139817.

[51] **Gerace C and Blndo C.** (2013) Reduplicative Paramnesia: Not Only One. Neuropsychaitry Online. 1 Jul 2013. https://doi.org/10.1176/appi.neuropsych.12030072

[52] **Whitworth H**. (2007) LBD Travelers Extraordinaire. Lewy Body Digest, 2007. Reference #99 in lbdtools.com/lbd-references.

[53] **Ferman, T**. (2005). Understanding Behavioral Changes in Dementia. https://www.lbda.org/content/understanding-behavioral-changes-dementia.

[54] **Woods D, et al.** The effect of therapeutic touch on behavioral symptoms and cortisol in persons with dementia. Forschende Komplementarmedizin 16 3 (2009): 181-9. Retrieved from: https://www.ncbi.nlm.nih.gov/pubmed/19657203

[55] **Mortimer S.** (2018) The Latest News in Cannabis Clinical Trials. BioSpace. Sep 28, 2018. https://www.biospace.com/article/the-latest-news-in-cannabis-clinical-trials/

[56] **Freeman J.** (2019) Does CBD Oil Really Help Treat Arthritis Pain? Oct. 4, 2019. RheumatoidArthritis Support Network. https://www.rheumatoidarthritis.org/cbd-oil/

[57] **Pines Education Institute**. (ongoing) Resources. Dementia Care Academy. https://dementiacareacademy.com/static/resources.htm.

[58] **Lewy Body Dementia Assn.** (ongoing) Local Support Groups. https://www.lbda.org/lbd-local-support-groups.

[59] **Family Caregiver Alliance**. Family Care Navigator. Phone: (800) 445.8106. Fax:(415)434.3508. Retrieved from: https://www.caregiver.org/family-care-navigator.

[60] **Preez J., et al**. (2018) The Role of Adult Day Services in Supporting the Occupational Participation of People with Dementia and Their Carers: An Integrative Review. Healthcare (Basel, Switzerland), 6(2), 43. doi:10.3390/healthcare6020043

[61] **Morrow A.** (2018) Palliative and Hospice Care for Dementia. How to Decide When Comfort Care Is Appropriate for a Loved One. Verywell Health and the Cleveland Clinic. May 30, 2018. https://www.verywellhealth.com/palliative-care-for-dementia-1132328

[62] **Alzheimer's Association** (2018) Medicare's hospice benefit for beneficiaries with Alzheimer's disease. Alzheimer's Association

webpage. https://www.alz.org/media/Documents/alzheimer's-dementia-medicare-hospice-benefit-ts.pdf

[63] **Galvin J., et. al.** (2010). Lewy body dementia: the caregiver experience of clinical care. Parkinsonism & related disorders, 16(6), 388-92. https://www.ncbi.nlm.nih.gov/pmc/articles/PMC2916037/

[64] **Lewy Body Journal**. (2003-2015) What are Lewy bodies? http://www.lewybodyjournal.org/whatlbdis.html.

[65] **Gibb, et. al.** (1987) Clinical And Pathological Features Of Diffuse Cortical Lewy Body Disease (Lewy Body Dementia). Brain, Vol. 110, No. 5, 961-1153, 1987. http://brain.oxfordjournals.org/cgi/content/abstract/110/5/961.

[66] **Jones E and Morrison J.**(1999) Cerebral Cortex, Volume 14. Neurodegenerative and Age-Related Changes in Structure and Function of Cerebral Cortex. Kluwer Academic/Plenum Publishers. New York. 1999.

[67] **McKeith I., et al.** (1996) Consensus guidelines for the clinical and pathologic diagnosis of dementia with Lewy bodies (DLB): Report of the consortium on DLB international workshop. Neurology. 1996; 47:196-1124. http://www.neurology.org/cgi/content/abstract/47/5/196.

[68] **ICD9Data.com.**(2008) Diagnosis 331.82. Dementia with Lewy bodies. http://www.icd9data.com/2008/Volume1/320-389/330-337/331/331.82.htm.

[69] **Lewy Body Society.** (2013) Dementia with Lewy Bodies receives formal recognition and classification. https://www.lewybody.org/dementia-with-lewy-bodies-receives-formal-recognition-and-classification/

[70] **Lippa C., et al**. (2007) DLB and PDD boundary issues. Diagnosis, treatment, molecular pathology, and biomarkers. Neurology 2007;68:812-819 © 2007 American Academy of Neurology. https://www.semanticscholar.org/paper/DLB-and-PDD-boundary-issues%3A-diagnosis%2C-treatment%2C-Lippa-Duda/579733a8573f3c6ed8e51bb9818981583b1deb73

[71] **Emre M., et al**. (2007) Clinical diagnostic criteria for dementia associated with Parkinson's disease. Mov Disord. 2007 Sep 15;22(12):1689-707; quiz 1837. https://www.semanticscholar.org/paper/Clinical-diagnostic-criteria-for-dementia-with-Emre-Aarsland/608e03d15fb37acbb745b776bbf3f87c855c1763.

[72] **McKeith, I. G., Boeve, B. F., Dickson, D. W., et. al.** (2017) Diagnosis and management of dementia with Lewy bodies: Fourth consensus report of the DLB Consortium. Neurology, 89(1), 88-100.

[73] **Surendranathan A and O'Brien J** (2018) Clinical imaging in dementia with Lewy bodies Evidence-Based Mental Health 2018;21:61-65. https://ebmh.bmj.com/content/21/2/61

[74] **Warr L and Walker Z.** (2012) Identification of biomarkers in Lewy-body disorders. Q J Nucl Med Mol Imaging. 2012 Feb;56(1):39-54. https://www.ncbi.nlm.nih.gov/pubmed/22460159

[75] **Odagiri H, et. al.** (2016) On the Utility of MIBG SPECT/CT in Evaluating Cardiac Sympathetic Dysfunction in Lewy Body Diseases. Plos One. April 7, 2016. doi.org/10.1371/journal.pone.0152746

[76] **Whitwell, J, et. al.** (2017) 18F-FDG PET in Posterior Cortical Atrophy and Dementia with Lewy Bodies. Journal of nuclear medicine: official publication, Society of Nuclear Medicine, 58(4), 632-638. https://www.ncbi.nlm.nih.gov/pmc/articles/PMC5373504/

[77] **Steinberg M and Lyketsos C.** (2012). Atypical Antipsychotic Use In Patients With Dementia: Managing Safety Concerns. The American Journal of Psychiatry, 169(9), 900–906. http://doi.org/10.1176/appi.ajp.2012.12030342

* 9 7 8 0 9 9 1 6 4 8 8 9 4 *